Optimized Healthcare: Leveraging Technology for Efficiency and Accessibility

(Part 2)

Edited by

Akhil Sharma
R. J. College of Pharmacy
Raipur, Gharbara, Tappal, Khair
Uttar Pradesh 202165, India

Shaweta Sharma
School of Medical and Allied Sciences
Galgotias University Yamuna Expressway
Gautam Buddha Nagar Uttar Pradesh 201310
India

Pankaj Kumar Singh
Institute of Biomedicine University
of Turku, Turku, Finland

&

Neeraj Kumar Fuloria
Department of Pharmaceutical Chemistry
Faculty of Pharmacy, AIMST University
Semeling Campus, Jalan Bedong–Semeling
08100 Bedong, Kedah Darul Aman, Malaysia

Optimized Healthcare: Leveraging Technology for Efficiency and Accessibility (Part 2)

Editors: Akhil Sharma, Shaweta Sharma, Pankaj Kumar Singh & Neeraj Kumar Fuloria

ISBN (Online): 979-8-89881-159-4

ISBN (Print): 979-8-89881-160-0

ISBN (Paperback): 979-8-89881-161-7

Published by Bentham Science Publishers Pte. Ltd. Singapore, in collaboration with Eureka Conferences, USA. All Rights Reserved.

First published in 2025.

need for a court order if at any point you breach any terms of this License Agreement. In no event will any delay or failure by Bentham Science Publishers in enforcing your compliance with this License Agreement constitute a waiver of any of its rights.

3. You acknowledge that you have read this License Agreement, and agree to be bound by its terms and conditions. To the extent that any other terms and conditions presented on any website of Bentham Science Publishers conflict with, or are inconsistent with, the terms and conditions set out in this License Agreement, you acknowledge that the terms and conditions set out in this License Agreement shall prevail.

Bentham Science Publishers Pte. Ltd.
No. 9 Raffles Place
Office No. 26-01
Singapore 048619
Singapore
Email: subscriptions@benthamscience.net

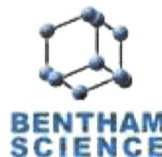

**BENTHAM
SCIENCE**

CONTENTS

Shaweta Sharma, Akhil Sharma, Sunita, Akanksha Sharma, Ashish Verma and
Geetika Goel

Shaweta Sharma, Akhil Sharma, Ashish Verma, Akanksha Sharma and Rakesh Patel

FOREWORD

In "Optimized Healthcare: Leveraging Technology for Efficiency and Accessibility," the book embarks on a journey into the future of healthcare, where the fusion of technology and innovation promises to reshape the landscape of patient care. This book arrives at a critical juncture in the evolution of healthcare as the demand for enhanced efficiency and accessibility reaches unprecedented levels. Against this backdrop, the exploration of how technology can be leveraged to meet these challenges is both timely and essential. Through insightful analyses, real-world examples, and forward-thinking strategies, this book illuminates the transformative potential of digital innovations such as data analytics, telemedicine, and artificial intelligence. By embracing these tools and fostering collaboration across the healthcare ecosystem, we can chart a path toward a more efficient, accessible, and patient-centric healthcare system. The book "Optimized Healthcare," gives an advantage to lead constructive change and create a future in which technology enables to provide everyone with better care.

Shivkanya Fuloria
Department of Pharmaceutical Chemistry
Faculty of Pharmacy, AIMST University
Semeling Campus, Jalan Bedong–Semeling
08100 Bedong, Kedah Darul Aman, Malaysia

PREFACE

The book "Optimized Healthcare: Leveraging Technology for Efficiency and Accessibility" emerges at a pivotal moment in the evolution of healthcare, where the integration of technology holds the key to addressing the complex challenges facing healthcare systems worldwide. In this preface, the book embarks on a journey into the heart of this convergence, exploring how digital innovations can revolutionize healthcare delivery to enhance efficiency and accessibility. Through a comprehensive examination of technologies such as data analytics, telemedicine, artificial intelligence, and digital health platforms, it uncovers transformative opportunities to streamline processes, improve care coordination, and personalize patient experiences. Moreover, the book delves into the ethical considerations and practical strategies essential for harnessing the full potential of technology while ensuring equitable access and patient-centered care. As we embark on this exploration, let us seize the opportunity to optimize healthcare for the benefit of individuals and communities around the globe.

Akhil Sharma
R. J. College of Pharmacy
Raipur, Gharbara, Tappal, Khair
Uttar Pradesh 202165, India

Shaweta Sharma
School of Medical and Allied Sciences
Galgotias University Yamuna Expressway
Gautam Buddha Nagar Uttar Pradesh 201310
India

Pankaj Kumar Singh
Institute of Biomedicine University
of Turku, Turku, Finland

&

Neeraj Kumar Fuloria
Department of Pharmaceutical Chemistry
Faculty of Pharmacy, AIMST University
Semeling Campus, Jalan Bedong–Semeling
08100 Bedong, Kedah Darul Aman, Malaysia

List of Contributors

Ashish Verma	Mangalmay Pharmacy College, Greater Noida, Uttar Pradesh 201306, India
Akhil Sharma	R.J. College of Pharmacy, Raipur, Gharbara, Tappal, Khair, Uttar Pradesh 202165, India
Akanksha Sharma	R.J. College of Pharmacy, Raipur, Gharbara, Tappal, Khair, Uttar Pradesh 202165, India
Geetika Goel	Motherhood University, Village Karoundi, Bhagwanpur, Roorkee, Uttarakhand 247661, India
Mohammad Mansoor	Devaki Amma Memorial College of Pharmacy, Chelembra, Mallapuram, Kerala 673634, India
Neeraj Kumar Fuloria	Department of Pharmaceutical Chemistry, Faculty of Pharmacy, AIMST University, Semeling Campus, Jalan Bedong-Semeling, Bedong, Kedah Darul Aman, Malaysia-08100, India
Pankaj Kumar Singh	Institute of Biomedicine University of Turku, Turku, Finland
P. Syamjith	Devaki Amma Memorial College of Pharmacy, Chelembra, Mallapuram, Kerala 673634, India
Rakesh Patel	Malwa Institute of Pharmaceutical Science, Indore, Madhya Pradesh 452001, India
Shaweta Sharma	School of Medical and Allied Sciences, Galgotias University, Gautam Buddha Nagar, Uttar Pradesh 201310, India
Swati Mutha	School of Pharmacy, Vishwakarma University, Pune, Maharashtra 411002, India
Satyabrata Bhanja	RITEE College of Pharmacy, NH-6, Chhatauna, Mandir Hasaud, Raipur, Chhattisgarh 492001, India
Sunita	R.J. College of Pharmacy, Raipur, Gharbara, Tappal, Khair, Uttar Pradesh 202165, India
Zeba Siddiqui	Amity Institute of Pharmacy, Amity University, Gwalior, Madhya Pradesh 474005, India

CHAPTER 1

Mobile Health Solutions for Accessibility

Swati Mutha[1], Ashish Verma[2], Akhil Sharma[3], Akanksha Sharma[3], Pankaj Kumar Singh[4] and Shaweta Sharma[5,*]

[1] *School of Pharmacy, Vishwakarma University, Pune, Maharashtra 411002, India*

[2] *Mangalmay Pharmacy College, Greater Noida, Uttar Pradesh 201306, India*

[3] *R.J. College of Pharmacy, Raipur, Gharbara, Tappal, Khair, Uttar Pradesh 202165, India*

[4] *Institute of Biomedicine University of Turku, Turku, Finland*

[5] *School of Medical and Allied Sciences, Galgotias University, Yamuna Expressway, Gautam Buddha Nagar, Uttar Pradesh 201310, India*

Abstract: The advancements in mobile devices, sensors, and other technologies have transformed mHealth into a wide-ranging and cost-effective platform that justifies its value as the bridge for gaps in current health service delivery. This chapter gives a detailed concept of mHealth solutions and highlights the innovations towards improved access to healthcare among underprivileged and remote communities. The chapter delves into key elements of mHealth, including mobile devices, sensor technologies, health applications, and AI assistants, and examines how connectivity will help improve the accessibility of mHealth. It discusses the key technologies behind mHealth, such as mobile applications, wearable devices, telemedicine platforms, and digital health records. It provides insights into how these technologies are used to enhance healthcare outcomes. It also describes the use of mHealth to manage chronic diseases, address mental health issues, and provide maternal and child health services and disability services. It also explores potential mechanisms through which the mHealth landscape empowers patients through enhanced engagement, increased health literacy, and patient-centred care methods. Despite its many benefits, the chapter addresses challenges in implementing mHealth solutions, particularly concerning the digital divide, infrastructure limitations, and privacy concerns.

Keywords: Healthcare accessibility, Health apps, mHealth, Mobile health technologies, Patient empowerment, Wearable devices.

INTRODUCTION

Mobile Health, commonly referred to as mHealth, encompasses the use of mobile devices, wireless technologies, and digital applications to support healthcare

* **Corresponding author Shaweta Sharma:** School of Medical and Allied Sciences, Galgotias University, Yamuna Expressway, Gautam Buddha Nagar, Uttar Pradesh 201310, India; E-mail: shawetasharma@galgotiasuniversity.edu.in

practices, services, and information sharing. Its diverse functions encompass remote patient monitoring, telemedicine consultations, health education initiatives, and chronic disease management programs. By capitalising on the widespread adoption of mobile gadgets, mHealth endeavours to bridge the divide between providers and patients, especially those in underserved areas. Its remit additionally involves collecting health-related information, personalised interventions, and incorporating artificial intelligence for predictive evaluation, cementing its role as a foundation of contemporary medical systems [1, 2].

Evolution of mHealth Technologies

The progression of mHealth is deeply intertwined with innovations in mobile communication technologies and the spread of smartphones. Early applications of mHealth were basic, focusing primarily on SMS-based health awareness campaigns and appointment reminders. The debut of wearable devices capable of tracking vital signs such as heart rate, blood pressure, and glucose levels marked a significant leap forward. The incorporation of cloud computing and 5G connectivity further expanded mHealth's abilities, enabling real-time data transmission and more robust telemedicine platforms. Recent years have borne witness to the inclusion of artificial intelligence (AI) and machine learning into mHealth applications, enhancing diagnostic precision and fostering personalised healthcare. This continuous evolution reflects mHealth's potential to reshape how healthcare is delivered and accessed globally [3 - 5].

Impact of mHealth on Healthcare Delivery

The impact of mHealth on healthcare delivery is genuinely transformative, addressing long-standing challenges involving accessibility, affordability, and efficiency. By facilitating remote consultations, mHealth reduces the necessity for in-person visits, mainly benefiting patients in rural or underserved areas. This not only saves time and costs but also alleviates the strain on healthcare infrastructure. Meanwhile, mHealth empowers patients with tools for self-monitoring and management of chronic conditions, fostering a proactive approach towards health. For healthcare providers, mHealth offers streamlined communication as well as coordination, enabling better decision-making and enhanced patient outcomes [6, 7].

During times of public health crises, mHealth has proved invaluable in disseminating information, tracking infections, and maintaining continuity of care. Despite challenges such as data security as well as technology access disparities, the adoption of mHealth continues to grow, paving the path for a more connected and efficient healthcare ecosystem. By encompassing these facets, mHealth stands at the forefront of digital transformation in healthcare, providing pioneering solutions that improve patient care as well as operational efficiencies while also using language varying in complexity from simple to more sophisticated terms [8, 9].

MOBILE HEALTH AND ACCESSIBILITY

Mobile health technologies promise to transform medical care by boosting access, engaging patients, and tackling disparities. Technologies like smartphones, wearables, and telehealth offer creative solutions to link those in places lacking customary clinics to critical care. By capitalising on apps, gadgets, and networks, mHealth aims to make treatment available to more individuals while allowing them to influence their well-being. Some tools distribute health information, while others enable remote monitoring and virtual consultations. Progress depends on addressing digital divides and ensuring privacy. Overall, these evolving platforms could help everybody obtain quality care wherever needed. Fig. (**1**) describes the critical role of mHealth in improving healthcare accessibility [10, 11].

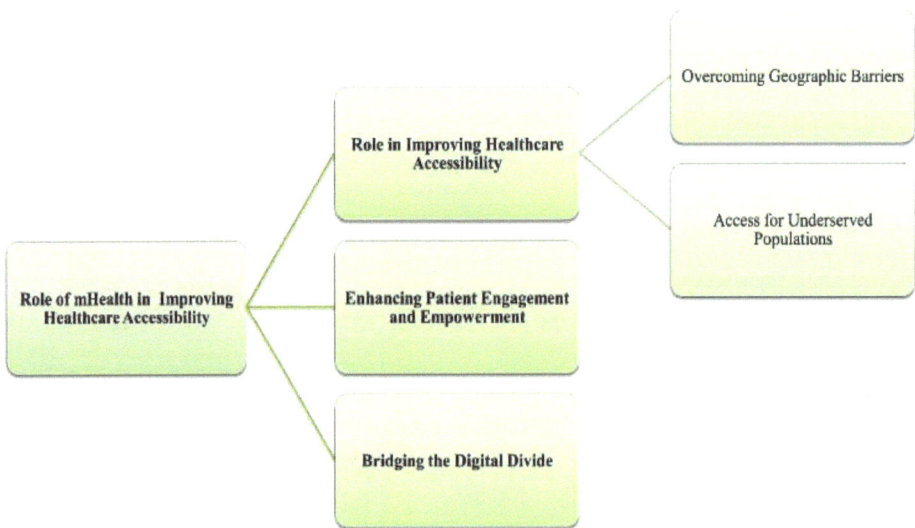

Fig. (1). Role of mHealth in improving healthcare accessibility.

Role in Improving Healthcare Accessibility

The role of mHealth in the improvement of accessibility of the healthcare system is discussed below.

Overcoming Geographic Barriers

Among the many contributions of mHealth, few compare to its ability to help break geographic boundaries that make it difficult to deliver healthcare. Healthcare facilities and skilled personnel are often sparse, which leaves populations in remote areas unable to receive treatment in a timely manner. The standard solution for this challenge is mHealth, which allows mobile phones for virtual consultation, telemonitoring, and digital prescriptions. Telemedicine, where a rural patient can consult with a specialist based in an urban centre without having to travel to that specialist, saves costs and time. Similarly, mHealth tools enable the adequate collection and transmission of health data in order to monitor patients remotely and provide continuous care by clinicians [12, 13].

Access for Underserved Populations

Underserved populations, including low-income groups and marginalised communities, often face significant barriers to healthcare access. These challenges consist of financial limitations, language obstacles, and cultural stigmas. mHealth interventions focus on these groups by providing affordable interventions through mobile phones and smartphones. For instance, SMS services to circulate health knowledge have been successful in increasing the health literacy of poor groups. Moreover, mHealth applications tailored to local languages and cultural contexts can further reduce disparities, ensuring healthcare inclusivity [14, 15].

Enhancing Patient Engagement and Empowerment

Mobile health (mHealth) promotes patient engagement through its tools, helping an individual become proactive about their health. Real-time access to patient health provides mobile apps for fitness, diet, medication compliance, chronic disease management, and more. These tools promote prevention-based health habits and make prudent choices among other people. Additionally, patient portals provide ways to view medical records, book appointments, and message healthcare providers, thus making the patient more in control and more of a partner in their health. Treatment adherence and maintenance of a healthy lifestyle enable patients to achieve better outcomes [16, 17].

Bridging the Digital Divide

Despite its potential, the digital divide remains a critical challenge for mHealth initiatives. Users of mHealth see aggregated data, and providers see disaggregated data from their services. Bridging this divide is key to driving equal access to healthcare. By investing in low-cost technologies, expanding internet access, and offering digital literacy programs, governments, NGOs, and the private sector are crucial in bridging this divide. Offline functionality and low-cost devices can help extend the reach of the health service to digitally excluded populations [18, 19].

ELEMENTS OF MOBILE HEALTH

The key components of mHealth can be categorised into three main areas: hardware, software, and connectivity. Each of these elements plays a pivotal role in the effective functioning of mHealth systems, which have become essential tools in modern healthcare. The three main components of mobile health are represented in Fig. (**2**).

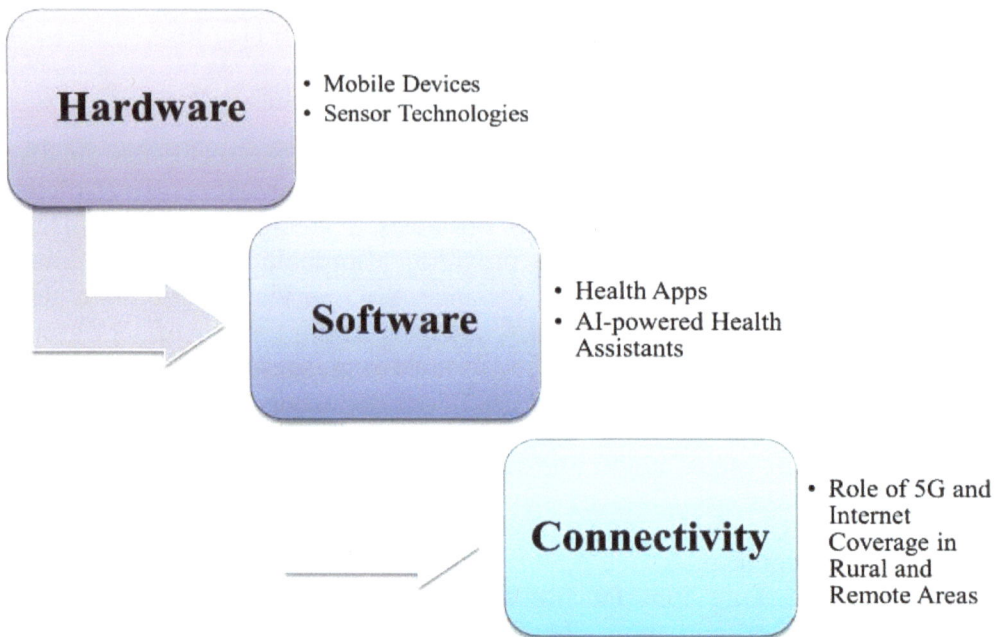

Fig. (2). Elements of mHealth.

Hardware

Hardware is the fundamental layer for any mHealth solution that is necessary in order to gather data, interact with patients, and monitor them in real-time. Mobile phones, tablets, and wearables are the primary devices that enable mHealth participation. This includes the use of smartphones and tablets for health data management, accessing health-related data, and connecting with health care providers *via* telemedicine platforms. These wearable devices, many of which come in the accessories of smartwatches, fitness trackers, and dedicated medical wearables, provide real-time information about health standards with the ability to monitor various parameters such as vital signs, physical activity, and work conditions, and monitoring of sleep details, among others. These devices offer critical information for continuous health monitoring, chronic disease management, and preventive care [20, 21].

Integrated sensor technologies, such as those embedded in wearable devices and mobile hardware, are critical to increasing the utility and precision of mHealth. Sugar detectors for diabetes, cardiac monitoring devices, heart feel sensors, and blood pressure detectors are utility tools for advancement and active well-being keepers. With these sensors, patients and healthcare professionals can monitor health metrics accurately, encouraging better decision-making and timely interventions. Improvements in sensors are increasing the sensitivity, specificity, and comfort of these instruments, and new application domains for remote monitoring of health [22, 23].

Software

Leading mHealth solutions are equally dependent on the software applications that deliver the tools enabling users to control, interpret, and utilise their health data. Health apps encompass a broad range of functionality, including fitness, medication reminders, diagnostics, and appointment management systems. These applications enable users to monitor their daily health habits, track disease progression, and share data with healthcare providers. Leading mHealth solutions are equally dependent on the software applications that deliver the tools enabling users to control, interpret, and utilise their health data. Health apps encompass a broad range of functionality, including fitness, medication reminders, diagnostics, and appointment management systems [24, 25].

Artificial Intelligence (AI) is another critical software component in the mHealth ecosystem. For instance, AI-powered health assistants use machine learning algorithms to analyse large datasets and provide personalised health recommendations. They can help patients diagnose, suggest healthy behaviour changes, or manage chronic disease. It can improve the overall efficacy of healthcare by aiding decisions made regarding diagnostics, treatment strategies, and tailored care pathways. In addition, AI can reduce the burden on healthcare professionals through the automation of routine tasks such as booking an appointment, patient triage, and follow-up reminders [26, 27].

AI-driven mHealth tools are also revolutionising the analysis and interpretation of healthcare data. Advanced analytics enables automation of real-time decision-making and pattern identification from datasets too big for a human practitioner to parallel process. Big data, combined with AI, can be used to analyse patient information contained in a range of sources, including wearable devices and lab results, to predict health outcomes and identify possible risks. This is an actionable insight that can be turned into proactive care, and healthcare providers can address complications or diseases before they progress to a critical state [28, 29].

Connectivity

The critical characteristic that is essential for mHealth solutions is connectivity, which allows communication to take place from healthcare providers to patients and between various healthcare systems. The importance of resilient, high-speed connectivity cannot be overemphasised, as it assures seamless data transmission of health information, real-time monitoring, and optimised delivery of remote healthcare services [30]. 5G is one of the areas most impacted by connectivity for mHealth solutions. 5G networks offer greater bandwidth, reduced latency, and higher reliability, which means they can transfer data more quickly and efficiently, and this is very important for remote health monitoring and telemedicine. 5G enables healthcare providers to provide better interactive and responsive services in 5G-enabled smart hospitals, including real-time video consultation, remote surgery, and remote monitoring of chronic patients [31].

5G has mHealth application areas, which are not limited to urban settings. However, 5G will help bridge the digital divide by allowing high-quality healthcare services to be offered in remote and rural areas where access to healthcare is already limited. In these areas, the internet is often unstable, and health resources are scarce, creating a gap that prevents patients from obtaining medical assistance promptly. Telemedicine, remote consultations, and health education programs can be enabled through the availability of 5G networks in these areas, improving access to healthcare and potentially helping to reduce disparities. Moreover, as connectivity is enhanced, the sharing of data, in most cases, takes place in real time between healthcare service providers, improving collaboration and enabling doctors to provide the best care possible to their patients no matter where the patients are located [32, 33].

5G enables increased use of mHealth, but it also helps with the expanded use of IoT (Internet of Things) devices in health care in general. Devices for the Internet of Things, like smart thermometers, wearable glucose monitors, and heart rate monitors, can send health data to be analysed and decided by a cloud-based platform, requiring constant and fast internet connectivity. The volume and speed capability of data transmission in 5G networks can accommodate the growing number of IoT devices in healthcare, thus facilitating more complex and scalable health monitoring [34, 35].

TECHNOLOGIES DRIVING MOBILE HEALTH

Several key technologies are driving the success of mHealth solutions, including mobile applications, wearable devices, telemedicine platforms, remote monitoring systems, and the integration of electronic health records (EHR) [36].

Mobile Applications

Mobile health (mHealth) solutions are represented mainly by mobile applications that have the potential to be a groundbreaking new way of providing access to healthcare. These are apps for smartphones, tablets, and other handheld devices with a wide range of functionality targeting healthcare needs, from monitoring of patients to health education. Their strength is their ability to integrate into healthcare systems, be combined with wearables, and form other digital health tools to form a larger ecosystem that supports both the patient and the healthcare provider [37].

The usage of fitness and wellness applications has become typical for advocating a healthy lifestyle. These apps also integrate closely with wearables to go beyond counting steps to more advanced metrics such as physical activity, sleep patterns, and heart rate, ultimately enhancing users' emotional and physical health. In addition to mainly physical health, mental health apps provide many guided meditations, address cognitive behavioural therapy exercises, provide access to virtual counsellors, and reduce the rising concerns of mental well-being in the modern world [38].

Mobile apps facilitate clinical workflows and decision-making for health providers. Decision-support apps that use artificial intelligence evaluate patient data in order to help diagnose conditions and recommend treatments to patients. EHR apps also allow doctors to view patient-related information from anywhere, leading to greater efficiency and fewer mistakes. This functionality enhances the quality of care and lowers the cost of care by decreasing avoidable hospital visits and procedures [39].

One of the most significant benefits of mobile apps in mHealth is their role in health education and awareness. Public health applications broadcast disease, immunisation, and epidemic response information. In the case of the COVID-19 pandemic, such apps have been central to processes including contact tracing, symptom tracking, and dissemination of reliable information, highlighting the capacity of this technology to support global health crises [40].

Wearable Devices

Wearable devices have emerged as an integral component of mobile health (mHealth) solutions, fundamentally altering the landscape of traditional healthcare service delivery and monitoring. Wearable devices are specially made for users to wear, which help with real-time data collection, monitoring, and transmission to help exponential patient engagement and offer essential insights to healthcare professionals. These are biosensors, medical-grade wearables, smartwatches, *etc.*, and they are embedded with advanced sensors that can track a wide range of physiological parameters. This constant tracking of these parameters enables timely interventions, thus avoiding acute medical events and decreasing hospital readmission [41, 42].

A significant factor adding to the rise of wearable devices in mHealth solutions is progress in sensor technology, miniaturisation, and wireless communication. Most of these devices use Bluetooth, Wi-Fi, or cellular capabilities to send data directly to a smartphone, tablet, or cloud platform for seamless integration with existing healthcare systems. It also helps to reduce the burden of remote patient monitoring, *i.e.*, tracking a patient's health status while being miles apart from the patient's healthcare providers. Such devices can alert both patient and provider to changes in levels of blood sugar, such as wearable glucose monitors used for continuous glucose monitoring (CGM) for diabetic patients [43, 44].

These also facilitate the promotion of personalised health management as an aspect of the growing trend of increasing the popularity of wearable devices. This new set of data is constantly inputted based on an individual's health status, giving wearables the ability to detect personal habits, exercise routines, and sleeping habits, ultimately providing the illusion of advice for health decisions. Further, deep learning algorithms and ML advancements incorporated into these devices improve their predictive powers so that they can recognise patterns and anticipate problems before they become serious [45].

Telemedicine Platforms

Telemedicine, the use of telecommunications technology to provide healthcare services remotely, has become one of the most significant advancements in mHealth. Telemedicine platforms allow for real-time consultations between patients and healthcare providers, overcoming geographical and logistical barriers that often limit access to medical care, especially in rural and underserved populations. Telemedicine platforms enable patients to receive diagnoses, recommendations for treatment, and follow-up care using video conferencing, mobile apps, or other digital communication [46].

By allowing clinicians to triage non-urgent cases remotely, these platforms also help reduce the burden on healthcare settings. This improves the efficiency of the health care system, enabling clinical staff to reserve in-person visits for more urgent conditions while continuing to care for less urgent issues. Additionally, telemedicine allows continuing care whereby patients are able to interact with their healthcare providers regularly without travelling long distances, thus enhancing adherence to treatment [47].

Similarly, telemedicine platforms are adapting to advances in artificial intelligence (AI) and machine learning (ML), which may help healthcare providers automate some administrative tasks, ensure greater diagnostic accuracy, and even predict treatment outcomes. Such capabilities enable the integration of hospitalisation and help in telemedicine practices, facilitating added personalisation and effectiveness of care transmission [48].

Remote Monitoring Systems

Remote monitoring systems (RMS) are another critical mHealth-driving technology that enables the monitoring of patients' health conditions outside of traditional healthcare settings through the use of mobile health technologies. As an alternative to hospitalisation, remote monitoring uses wearable technology, sensors, and mobile apps to track valuable real-time data related to a patient's vital signs, chronic conditions, medication adherence, and other health metrics. It facilitates real-time monitoring, especially in the case of patients with chronic diseases, without the need for frequent visits to the healthcare facility [49].

Such systems are necessary for early detection and intervention. Remote monitoring systems can gather data on many health parameters and be used to notify healthcare providers when abnormalities or changes in a patient's condition indicate deterioration. For instance, RMS can monitor heart rate and blood pressure in patients suffering from cardiovascular diseases. It is able to notify the patient as well as the health care provider when there is a worrisome trend, which facilitates timely interventions to avert complications or hospitalisation [50].

They improve the quality of care but also reinforce patient empowerment by allowing people to take active control of their health. Patients track their health data *via* mobile apps or connected devices, improving self-awareness and participation in their treatment plans. That sense of ownership can strengthen compliance with prescribed therapies and lifestyle changes, both of which are critical in the management of chronic disease. In addition to this, RMS is also a key player in cutting healthcare costs. These systems can substantially reduce costs for patients and healthcare systems by minimising unnecessary doctor visits and hospital readmissions through continuous monitoring. Additionally, they play a part in the optimisation of healthcare resources since medical practitioners are able to take care of patients needing immediate help while remotely managing other patients and making the flow of work more manageable [51, 52].

Electronic Health Records (EHR) Integration in mHealth

The use of Electronic Health Records (EHR) by mHealth (mobile health) solutions is a significant paradigm shift in the current healthcare landscape. An EHR contains the medical and treatment history of a patient and is more expansive than an individual record, as it is a digital population of a patient's notes from multiple healthcare providers and clinical encounters. The fact that all affected data are digitalised makes it much easier to save, recover, and transmit patient information compared to traditional paper-based records. Coupled with EHRs, mHealth applications improve healthcare service delivery *via* improved data availability, continuity of care, and patient engagement [53, 54].

To the mHealth solution, one of the significant benefits of EHR integration is enhanced accessibility of data. Cloud infrastructure enables medical professionals to securely retrieve patient information across locations, dismantling geographic and organisational silos. This is especially important for telemedicine and remote monitoring scenarios, where physicians may have to assess patients in real-time and not *via* in-person visits. A patient with a chronic illness, for instance, who is receiving care in a rural or underserved area, could be monitored from remote locations, with data on the patient being shared with specialists in other institutions, resulting in faster diagnoses and improved outcomes. In addition, mHealth apps with integration to EHRs can enable the patient to self-manage by having real-time access to their medical history, lab results, medication record, and appointment schedule, which can encourage the patient to be active in their healthcare [55, 56].

Another essential advantage of EHRs is the continuity between different healthcare settings. Given the reality that patients may interact with numerous providers, such as primary care physicians, specialists, and emergency departments, the ability to access important information about a patient in one location is critical, which is where EHRs come into play. This minimises the risk of medical errors, test redundancy, and harmful drug interactions because healthcare providers have access to complete, current patient data. To give an example, a mobile app linked with EHRs can immediately remind physicians regarding modifications in patients' medical routines or send alerts regarding upcoming check-ups so that treatments are not missed, which can help in achieving better health status for the patients [57, 58].

With the integration of EHRs, mHealth applications can extend their functionalities to more personalised healthcare. Based on the data within the EHR, Mobile apps can provide targeted health recommendations, medication reminders, and lifestyle modifications based on the patient's condition. These recommendations can be improved even more with artificial intelligence (AI) and machine learning algorithms studying the patterns and trends associated with the overall patient treatment data. For example, based on the holistic health information chronologically collected in the EHR, mHealth tools can be developed with personalised health management functions, such as tailored exercise programs or diet information modules [59, 60].

HEALTHCARE APPS FOR WELLNESS AND MEDICAL SUPPORT

Table **1** represents popular mobile applications designed to assist users in various aspects of health management. These apps are available across different platforms like iOS and Android, offering features tailored to both personal wellness and clinical support for healthcare professionals.

Table 1. Various mobile applications designed for monitoring health.

S. No.	Apps Name	Purpose	Features	Platform
1	MyFitnessPal [61]	Dietary tracking and physical fitness	Food diary, exercise tracker, and calorie counter.	iOS, Android
2	Medisafe [62]	Medication management	Pill reminders, medication tracker, and dosage management.	iOS, Android
3	Teladoc Health [63]	Virtual consultations and telemedicine	Online doctor visits and online mental health support.	iOS, Android
4	Apple Health [64]	Health and wellness data integration	Exercise monitoring, health record storage, and ECG monitoring.	iOS
5	Epocrates [65]	Clinical decision support (CDS) for healthcare professionals	Drug interaction checker, medical calculators, and disease guides.	iOS, Android
6	Samsung Health [66]	Managing fitness and wellness	Monitor step count, stress levels monitoring, and sleep tracking.	Android
7	Ada Health [67]	AI-powered symptom checker	Individualised health assessment, and symptom tracking.	iOS, Android

ENHANCING HEALTHCARE THROUGH THE APPLICATION OF MOBILE HEALTH

With the increasing ubiquity of mobile devices, mHealth has become an essential component in the delivery of effective care, from chronic disease management, mental health support, maternal and child health, to disability support, teleconsultation, and virtual healthcare services. mHealth solutions have transformational capabilities across different domains of healthcare by allowing real-time monitoring, increasing accessibility to patients, and involving them in participatory care [68]. The application of mHealth in enhancing the healthcare system is summarised in Fig. (3).

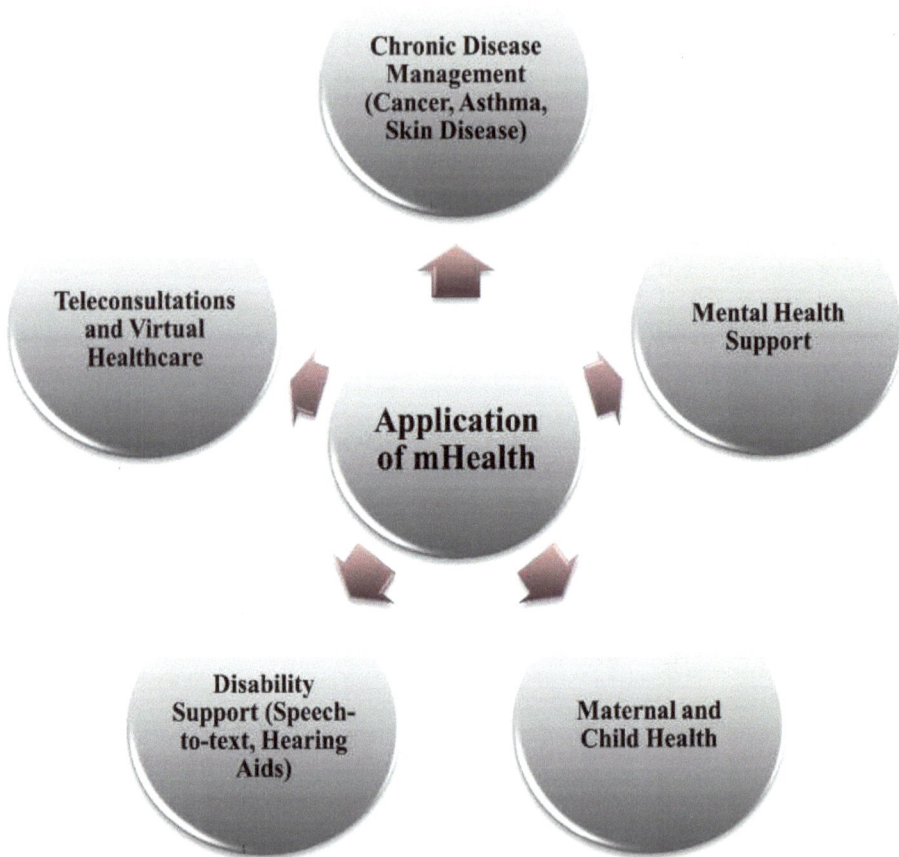

Fig. (3). Application of mHealth enhancing healthcare system.

mHealth in Chronic Disease Management

It helps manage chronic diseases such as cancer, asthma, and skin diseases. mHealth tools have also helped in the management and outcomes of these conditions *via* real-time monitoring, tailored care, and direct communication between patients and healthcare providers [69].

Cancer Management

Because cancer is a chronic disease and one of the leading global causes of death, it requires constant monitoring and management, which can be tiring for both patients and healthcare providers. mHealth applications are used for early detection, tracking of developed malignancies, and adherence to treatment in cancer care. The concept of wearable devices is not new, and there are many devices available today that can collect information about physiological activity, which provides essential data that may signal potential complications or side effects of treatment to care providers. In addition, applications for cancer patients enable patients to take charge of their medicines, schedule reminders for chemotherapy treatments, and report symptoms in real time, assisting in the anticipatory management of their conditions, thereby minimising routine hospital usage [70].

In addition, mHealth platforms facilitate better communication between patients and oncologists. Telemedicine capabilities provide the ability to consult virtually, overcoming the logistical barriers of transportation, which are exacerbated in patients in a rural or resource-poor setting. mHealth has even extended to mental health resources for cancer patients to alleviate the mental agony that comes with the disease. Incorporating these various technologies, mHealth applications aim to be patient-centred and deliver a more comprehensive strategy for cancer treatment, leading to enhanced therapeutic results and quality of life [71].

Asthma Management

Asthma is a global chronic lung disease that impacts millions of people and tends to require constant management, and flare-ups and severe attacks are entirely avoided. The use of mHealth applications in asthma management allows patients to record their symptoms, medication intake, and environmental factors that may induce an asthma attack. Wearables, such as smart inhalers, should be used to monitor inhaler use and adherence to prescribed treatment regimens. They can also alert if the medication is missed, thus avoiding the exacerbations that require hospitalisations [72].

Besides medication management, the mHealth app can also give real-time updates on environmental triggers, such as pollen levels and air quality, which can help asthma patients adapt their activities. Smartphone apps such as asthma and peak flow trackers aid in monitoring peak flow measurements in order for patients to keep an eye on lung function over time and provide early warning signs that can alert patients of an impending asthma attack. mHealth platforms facilitate remote monitoring and allow patients to be more involved and engaged in their health management, leading to reduced hospitalisations and improved disease control [73].

Skin Disease Management

Skin diseases and conditions (psoriasis, eczema, acne, *etc.*) are chronic. They can be debilitating and expensive to treat, necessitating continuous reinforcement to monitor and control flares, significantly affecting patients' quality of life. mHealth tools provide a structured approach to these chronic skin problems by providing a means for patients to collect daily reports of their symptoms, treatments, and triggers. Mobile applications for skin disease management allow patients to record their diseases *via* photo logs that could be sent to healthcare providers for offline evaluation. This reduces the need for in-person visits, which can be challenging for patients with mobility issues or those living in remote areas [74].

mHealth apps can provide information on lifestyle factors that contribute to flare-ups, for example, psoriasis or eczema, which are typically exacerbated by environmental triggers (*e.g.*, stress, temperature, and humidity). Such tools can offer personalised recommendations, for instance, in diet, stress management, or drug adjustments. In addition, mobile apps provide educational material; therefore, patients are more aware of their condition and eventually engage in better self-care, thus reducing flare-ups [75].

Wearable devices harness skin temperature, hydration level, and ultrasensitive ultraviolet (UV) exposure for skin disease management, too. Such devices can notify patients about possible triggers, giving them the opportunity to intervene before symptoms get worse. The mHealth applications combining real-time data collection and personalised recommendations can offer an essential advancement in the proactive management of chronic skin diseases, leading to better patient outcomes and quality of life [76].

Case Study of mHealth in Chronic Disease Management

In the treatment of chronic illnesses like cancer, asthma, and skin disorders, mobile health (mHealth) technologies have demonstrated outstanding potential.

Data of mHealth in Cancer Management

A comprehensive review and meta-analysis assessed how mHealth therapies affected cancer patients' health-related quality of life (HRQoL). The study comprised 25 studies with a total of 957 patients, including eight pre-post design studies and 17 randomised controlled trials. The most often researched mHealth therapies were mindfulness or stress management practices (3 studies), cognitive behavioural therapy (6 studies), and physical activity or fitness programs (9 studies). Improvements in cancer patients' HRQoL were linked to most of these therapies. The favourable impact of mHealth interventions on HRQoL was confirmed by the meta-analysis, indicating that these strategies have promise for improving cancer patients' quality of life [77].

Data of mHealth in Asthma Management

The features and impacts of mHealth apps made for asthma self-management were evaluated in a systematic study. Ten studies that assessed smartphone or tablet apps designed to enhance asthmatic patients' self-management results were included in the review. Clinical, patient-reported, and economic groups were used to classify the results. Five studies found that mHealth apps improved lung function, and two studies found that they improved asthma control. Two studies found no significant effect on self-efficacy scores, but three studies reported substantial increases in quality of life based on patient-reported outcomes. Economic results varied; some studies found that hospitalisations and medical visits had significantly decreased, while other studies found no discernible differences. Functionalities, including storing user-entered data, offering educational materials, and reminding patients, were standard in mHealth apps. When compared to conventional therapies, these multipurpose apps showed promise in improving asthma management and quality of life [78].

Data on mHealth in Skin Disease Management

The use of teledermatology, a subfield of mHealth, to treat skin conditions has grown, particularly in environments with limited resources. The usability and efficacy of the eSkinHealth mHealth app for diagnosing and treating skin-related neglected tropical diseases (skin NTDs) and other skin ailments in rural Côte d'Ivoire were assessed in mixed-methods pilot research. Over three months, the study included patients and local healthcare providers. Skin NTDs were recorded in 79 cases in the intervention group, which had the skin health app installed, compared to 17 cases in the control group. This difference was statistically significant (P =.002). Furthermore, 72.9% of cases in the intervention group had specific diagnoses entered into the app, while 66% of cases in the control group were simply recorded as "dermatosis" with no specific diagnosis. High user satisfaction was shown by the app's System Usability Scale (SUS) scores, which increased from 72.3 at baseline to 86.3 at the end of the trial. This study shows that in resource-constrained settings, mHealth apps such as Skin Health can improve skin disease identification and treatment [79].

The management of chronic illnesses like cancer, asthma, and skin disorders has been demonstrated to be improved by mHealth interventions. Particularly in situations when traditional healthcare resources are limited, these technologies provide easily accessible and efficient instruments for improving patient outcomes.

mHealth in Mental Health Support

Mobile health (mHealth) technologies have emerged as transformative tools in supporting mental health patients, enhancing real-time intervention in patients, and increasing accessibility to care. mHealth allows people to be treated for mental health conditions such as anxiety, depression, and stress using wearable sensors and mobile apps [80].

Accessibility and Reach

Perhaps the most pronounced benefit of using mHealth to support mental health is that it can transcend geographical and social divides. Numerous people struggle with mental health care in underserved or rural areas where access to actual care could meet their needs. The great potential of a mHealth application is that patients are given direct support, averting the need for an office visit and a long-term breaking of barriers (long waiting periods for appointments and travel costs). This broader accessibility is beneficial for marginalised populations that may really feel stigmatised or lack psychological well-being assets [81].

Precision Monitoring and Feedback

mHealth platforms allow real-time measurement of mental health status *via* embedded sensors and patient reports. These technologies offer real-time data to evaluate the mental well-being of the user by tracking their mood, sleep patterns, and physical activity (and other behavioural indicators). Apps like cognitive behavioural therapy (CBT), mood trackers, and stress management tools provide self-help strategies and immediate feedback, enabling users to be more proactive in their mental health care. The real-time observation effect yields regular management amid mental health disorders by tracking the potential warning signs and relapses beforehand [82, 83].

Personalised and Targeted Interventions

By tailoring mental health interventions to individual-specific needs, mHealth applications also offer a personalised approach to mental health care. Algorithms can then suggest customised recommendations for coping methods, relaxation approaches, or mental exercises based on the information provided by the user. This enables real-time adjustments made to the interventions based on user progress, providing feelings of agency and control over one's mental health journey. Furthermore, clinician mHealth tools may provide a window into the patient's condition, improving management and facilitating shared decision-making [84].

Reducing Stigma and Promoting Engagement

mHealth applications provide anonymity, which is extremely important, as stigma related to seeking mental health care is very prevalent. The combination of anonymity and ease of access can actually drive some people to seek help who may actively avoid regular care settings because of social phobia. In addition, the ease of use of the interface and gamification aspects of mHealth platforms encourage engagement and adherence that improve long-term outcomes regarding mental health support [85].

mHealth in Maternal and Child Health

Mobile health (mHealth) is a fast-growing field that introduces new ways to deliver maternal and child healthcare, increasing its availability, quality, and efficiency. For societies with little traditional healthcare infrastructure, mHealth platforms provide a lifeline, shoring up the interface between healthcare providers and patients. For maternal health, mHealth applications measure key parameters such as fetal development, maternal nutrition, and timing for prenatal care provision. By providing personalised reminders and educational content, these platforms motivate pregnant women to keep up with necessary health visits, vaccinations, and preventive screenings to minimise maternal morbidity and mortality [86].

Mobile apps that can provide access to health data in real time allow healthcare professionals to monitor high-risk pregnancies from a distance. This is especially important for women living in rural or underserved areas, where healthcare facilities may be few and far between. It is also beneficial for the early recognition of complications, which might become life-threatening, for the mother and child if not treated quickly, such as preeclampsia or gestational diabetes, through mobile-based tools. mHealth technologies reduce pregnancy and childbirth complications by improving prenatal care using mobile monitoring [87].

mHealth provides multiple functions regarding child health, *i.e.*, newborn care, vaccination, growth monitoring, *etc.* Custom apps for parents offer timely reminders about vaccination schedules and well-child visits, helping ensure that children get the vaccines and screening tests recommended for their age. This is especially advantageous in low-resource environments where providers may be in short supply. For example, mHealth solutions facilitate growth monitoring by supporting parents and caregivers in monitoring developmental milestones and identifying potential concerns at an early stage. mHealth applications provide access to health resources and expert advice on health care, allowing parents to make more informed decisions on their child's health [88].

Many mHealth platforms have educational content integrated into them that educates caregivers on how to identify danger signs in infants and toddlers as well as when the right time is to seek care. Such a solution can prove vital for the early detection of conditions like respiratory infections, malnutrition, or diarrhoea, which are common causes of child mortality in several low and middle-income countries. By increasing awareness and facilitating timely action, mHealth holds the promise of a substantial reduction of preventable maternal and child morbidity and mortality [89].

mHealth in Disability Support

Mobile health (mHealth) technologies have recently been recognised as either mobilising or potentially transformative within the disability domain. The most significant benefit of mHealth is that it can close accessibility gaps, providing solutions to allow people to understand their health and act upon it efficiently. mHealth applications can also be particularly important for the support of those who have speech or hearing impairments, making it easier for them to communicate, access services, and communicate with healthcare systems [90].

Speech-to-text apps are one of the more critical breakthroughs for anyone with a speech impairment or someone who cannot get their point across in the traditional way. Such apps transform spoken language into written text to improve communication with medical personnel, relatives, and the general public. Speech-to-text tools can also ensure information transfer is free from miscommunication, keeping accuracy intact and enhancing care delivery, especially for patients who may have impaired verbal communication, like people with speech disabilities, stroke survivors, and neurological disorders [91].

Hearing impairments that impact millions globally can be treated with mHealth technologies such as hearing aids, which have developed over the years with links to smartphones. Newer hearing aids can connect with mobile apps so users can adjust their hearing needs and receive immediate adjustments based on environmental factors. For example, people can change the volume, filter background noise, and customise sound settings using their smartphones by using apps. Additionally, mHealth-based solutions, such as video calls and captioned telemedicine services, enhance communication between patients with hearing impairments and healthcare providers, promoting better accessibility and healthcare engagement [92].

mHealth in Teleconsultations and Virtual Healthcare

Teleconsultations and virtual healthcare play a key role in healthcare transformation by addressing challenges like geographic isolation, healthcare availability, and wastage in health delivery. Teleconsultations, which constitute an essential part of mobile health (mHealth), can be defined as real-time consultations between patients and healthcare providers using digital technologies. This innovation takes healthcare to rural or unprivileged areas and has access to specialists that would not have been available otherwise. An example of this is where patients living in rural, remote, or lesser-developed low-income regions are able to consult with high-end top-tier doctors without travelling far away, which alleviates the burden of access disparities in health care [93]

The virtual healthcare field includes many telehealth services, not just teleconsultations but also remote patient monitoring, health tracking apps, and virtual health platforms. Such services allow healthcare providers to track patients' vital signs, chronic conditions, and treatment responses faster than with an in-person visit. Teleconsultations also provide convenience and flexibility, which can lead to enhanced patient satisfaction and compliance. It eliminates the travel and cost involved in a traditional visit by allowing patients to access healthcare services from home. Such convenience is especially valuable to patients who have difficulty with mobility, tight schedules, or chronic illness requiring regular follow-ups [94].

BENEFITS OF MOBILE HEALTH FOR ACCESSIBILITY

Mobile health (mHealth) is transforming accessibility by employing mobile technology to remove existing barriers to healthcare access. The inclusion of mHealth solutions opens up a variety of opportunities to make healthcare more affordable, patient-centred, and customisable, as well as improve health literacy more efficiently.

Cost-Effectiveness and Affordability

The most prominent benefit of mHealth is that it helps make healthcare more affordable and economical. Travel expenses, infrastructure needs, and the expense of medical personnel can make traditional healthcare systems too expensive, especially in underserved or remote areas. This is where mHealth platforms reduce these costs through virtual consultations, remote monitoring, and care provided through the power of mobile phones and devices. In particular, this could be impactful in rural or economically disadvantaged communities by minimising the necessity for patients to travel extended distances for essential examinations, diagnostic testing, and repeat treatment. Furthermore, mHealth applications enable cost-sharing between patients, healthcare providers, and insurers, leading to more affordable healthcare solutions. In some cases, preventative care offered *via* mHealth can help reduce the incidence of more severe conditions, ultimately lowering overall healthcare expenses by catching health issues early [95, 96].

Patient-Centric Care Models

mHealth enables patients to participate in self-health management by delivering a patient-centric care model. Traditional models would tend to put the healthcare provider at the centre of decision-making. Still, mHealth can empower patients to access their health data, track and monitor medicines *via* apps and devices, and manage their health and well-being. The result is higher-quality care that is better aligned with the patient's needs and preferences [97].

Patients can use mobile applications to remind themselves when to take medication, track their symptoms, and contact their healthcare provider while always having ownership over their health data. It is essential for patients with diseases where continued self-management is needed due to this shift to patient-centred models. Further, mobile health platforms enable personalised information transfer, delivering patient education, treatment options, and lifestyle recommendations relevant to a patient's health condition and treatment objectives [98].

Customisable and Scalable Solutions

A further critical advantage of mHealth is that it may deliver medical care that is highly tailored and scalable. Mobile health (mHealth) platforms can take into consideration the unique healthcare needs of various populations, ranging from individuals suffering from chronic diseases or the elderly to people living in remote regions. Mobile apps can be customised for certain conditions, which may include personalised exercise plans, dietary recommendations, mental health support, and medication reminders [99].

Due to the scalability and reach of mHealth systems to large populations, they provide unique advantages for public health interventions (vaccination campaigns or health education delivery). Since mHealth applications are primarily cloud-based, updating and upgrading features is super easy for healthcare providers, enabling them to stay more relevant and updated. Such scalability enables the addition of diverse health services, extending from preventive to specific health management, making the overall health system flexible and responsive to emerging demands [100].

Health Literacy Improvement

mHealth also plays a pivotal role in improving health literacy. Many individuals struggle to navigate complex healthcare systems or understand medical terminology, leading to a lack of engagement with their health. Mobile health apps provide simplified, easily consumable health information that allows users to make informed health decisions. Educational content in the form of instructional videos, articles, and interactive tools can organise information about understanding one's health condition, treatment options, and preventative measures in a way that is simplified and user-friendly [101].

For people with a low understanding of heterogeneous things about health, mHealth tools can close that gap by providing multilingual alternatives and visible aids. mHealth enhances health literacy and helps patients take greater ownership of their health, resulting in better health outcomes. Additionally, mobile platforms offer convenience by providing the ability to have information at all times and in all places, fostering continuous health promotion and healthcare engagement [102].

LIMITATIONS IN IMPLEMENTING MOBILE HEALTH

Since the accessibility, efficiency, and outcomes of mHealth can change the dynamic of healthcare delivery, the potential for positive impact is tremendous. But it has its drawbacks to execute. Such limitations are widespread in the technical, financial, regulatory, and social domains and must be overcome for the full potential of mHealth's benefits.

Technical Challenges

One of the critical challenges when employing mHealth solutions is their integration with existing healthcare systems. Mobile technologies are not integrated into existing healthcare infrastructures, which makes this model challenging to adopt. Moreover, the quality of health data collected from mobile devices will be questionable as factors such as the difference in the quality of the mobile device differs, and user compliance would have an impact on the quality of data. In addition, mHealth technologies often depend on the Internet and mobile networks, which may be unstable in rural or unserved areas, limiting the impact of these tools [103].

Privacy and Security Concerns

One of the significant limitations of mHealth is the potential threat to patient privacy and data security. Mobile health apps process closely related data and the risk of a data breach or unauthorised access is high where secrecy lacks force for health data. The absence of cybersecurity standards on multiple platforms makes the risk worse. The absence of clear and enforceable regulations can create a barrier such that patients may replace these technologies with a distinct reluctance to use them and healthcare providers with a reluctance to prescribe them [104].

Financial Barriers

Development, implementation, and maintenance of mHealth technologies can be prohibitively costly. Although the price of mobile devices is decreasing, implementing mHealth into healthcare systems requires substantial investment in infrastructure, training, and ongoing maintenance. These costs can represent a key hurdle for healthcare providers working in resource-limited settings. Additionally, reimbursement models for mHealth are still being developed, and most health insurers still do not reimburse mobile health interventions, which may represent an additional barrier to the adoption of mobile health [105].

User Engagement and Literacy

User engagement is a critical factor in the effectiveness of mHealth technologies. Most patients, especially older adults or those with limited digital literacy, may have difficulty using mobile health tools. This potentially hinders the uptake of mHealth, especially in populations who stand to benefit from it most. Furthermore, inequalities in smartphone and internet access among socioeconomic groups can worsen health inequities [106].

CONCLUSION

The use of mobile health (mHealth) solutions is a paradigm shift in the healthcare landscape, especially for providing healthcare services to marginalised and remote communities. With the tremendous growth of mobile technologies, healthcare delivery has also evolved to be more patient-centric, efficient, and flexible. The integration of mobile devices, sensor technologies, and health applications has enabled mHealth solutions to become an accessible health service platform for a broader population, especially in areas where traditional healthcare infrastructure is lacking.

Collectively, the main building blocks of mHealth address geographical and logistical barriers, allowing mHealth to be effectively delivered to patients within rural and underserved populations. Adding to this, AI-enabled health assistants and telemedicine platforms offer extra support, allowing people to engage more with their care and take charge of their health management.

mHealth technologies are used to improve the health outcomes of chronic diseases, mental health, maternal and child health, and disability support care through real-time monitoring and personalised care. By offering scalable and customisable solutions, mHealth promotes affordability and cost-effectiveness, making healthcare more accessible to those who need it most.

However, challenges such as the need for strong internet connectivity in rural areas, digital awareness of patients, and the incorporation of these technologies into currently functional healthcare systems still prevent successful implementation. Despite these limitations, the promise that mHealth has to reduce the digital divide and improve accessibility, engagement, and empowerment merits further investigation. As technology continues to evolve, mHealth will play an increasingly vital role in shaping the future of accessible, patient-centric healthcare globally.

CONSENT FOR PUBLICATON

All authors have given their consent for publication. The authors authorised Shaweta Sharma to handle all correspondences.

ACKNOWLEDGEMENTS

Authors are highly thankful to their Universities/Colleges for providing library facilities for the literature survey.

REFERENCES

[1]   Olla P, Shimskey C. mHealth taxonomy: a literature survey of mobile health applications. Health Technol (Berl) 2015; 4(4): 299-308.
[http://dx.doi.org/10.1007/s12553-014-0093-8]

[2]   Chahal BP, Sharma U, Bansal B. Innovative financing models and future directions in healthcare: Evaluating the impact of financial strategies on digital health outcomes and innovation In: Driving global health and sustainable development goals with smart technology. IGI Global Scientific Publishing 2025; pp. 267-302.

[3]   Fiordelli M, Diviani N, Schulz PJ. Mapping mHealth research: a decade of evolution. J Med Internet Res 2013; 15(5): e95.
[http://dx.doi.org/10.2196/jmir.2430] [PMID: 23697600]

[4]   Istepanian RS, AlAnzi T. Mobile health (m-health): Evidence-based progress or scientific retrogression. In: Feng DD, Ed. Biomedical information technology. 2nd ed. London: Academic Press. 2020; p. 717-733.

[5]   Mullachery B, Alismail S. A smart healthcare framework: opportunities for integrating emerging technologies (5G, IoT, AI, and GIS). In: Proceedings of the Future Technologies Conference. Cham: Springer International Publishing 2022; pp. 325-340.

[6]   Faiola A, Papautsky EL, Isola M. Empowering the ageing with mobile health: a mHealth framework for supporting sustainable healthy lifestyle behaviour. Curr Probl Cardiol 2019; 44(8): 232-66.
[http://dx.doi.org/10.1016/j.cpcardiol.2018.06.003] [PMID: 30185374]

[7] Mladin OA, Spinean A, Carniciu S, Serafinceanu C. The transformative power of mHealth apps: empowering patients with obesity and diabetes – a narrative review. J Med Life 2024; 17(12): 1030-5.
[http://dx.doi.org/10.25122/jml-2024-0340] [PMID: 39877040]

[8] Oloruntoba Babawarun , Babawarun O, Olorunsogo TO. Mobile health (health) innovations for public health feedback: a global perspective. Intl Med Sci Res J 2024; 4(3): 235-46.
[http://dx.doi.org/10.51594/imsrj.v4i3.915]

[9] Liaqat M, Mushtaq M, Jamil A, *et al.* Mobile health interventions: A frontier for mitigating the global burden of cardiovascular disease. Cureus 2024; 16(6): e62157.
[http://dx.doi.org/10.7759/cureus.62157] [PMID: 38993461]

[10] Mechael PN. The case for mHealth in developing countries. Innov (Camb, Mass) 2009; 4(1): 103-18.
[http://dx.doi.org/10.1162/itgg.2009.4.1.103]

[11] Istepanian RSH. Mobile health (m-Health) in retrospect: the known unknowns. Int J Environ Res Public Health 2022; 19(7): 3747.
[http://dx.doi.org/10.3390/ijerph19073747] [PMID: 35409431]

[12] Peprah P, Abalo EM, Agyemang-Duah W, *et al.* Lessening barriers to healthcare in rural Ghana: providers and users' perspectives on the role of mHealth technology. A qualitative exploration. BMC Med Inform Decis Mak 2020; 20(1): 27.
[http://dx.doi.org/10.1186/s12911-020-1040-4] [PMID: 32041608]

[13] El-Rashidy N, El-Sappagh S, Islam SMR, M El-Bakry H, Abdelrazek S. Mobile health in remote patient monitoring for chronic diseases: Principles, trends, and challenges. Diagnostics (Basel) 2021; 11(4): 607.
[http://dx.doi.org/10.3390/diagnostics11040607] [PMID: 33805471]

[14] van Veen T, Binz S, Muminovic M, *et al.* The potential of mobile health technology to reduce health disparities in underserved communities. West J Emerg Med 2019; 20(5): 799-802.
[http://dx.doi.org/10.5811/westjem.2019.6.41911] [PMID: 31539337]

[15] Déglise C, Suggs LS, Odermatt P. Short message service (SMS) applications for disease prevention in developing countries. J Med Internet Res 2012; 14(1): e3.
[http://dx.doi.org/10.2196/jmir.1823] [PMID: 22262730]

[16] Morley J, Floridi L. The limits of empowerment: how to reframe the role of mHealth tools in the healthcare ecosystem. Sci Eng Ethics 2020; 26(3): 1159-83.
[http://dx.doi.org/10.1007/s11948-019-00115-1] [PMID: 31172424]

[17] Hamine S, Gerth-Guyette E, Faulx D, Green BB, Ginsburg AS. Impact of mHealth chronic disease management on treatment adherence and patient outcomes: a systematic review. J Med Internet Res 2015; 17(2): e52.
[http://dx.doi.org/10.2196/jmir.3951] [PMID: 25803266]

[18] Michael P, Batavia H, Kaonga N, Searle S, Kwan A, Goldberger A, Fu L, Ossman J. Barriers and gaps affecting mHealth in low and middle-income countries: Policy white paper. 1970.

[19] Srivastava SC, Shainesh G. Bridging the service divide through digitally enabled service innovations. Manage Inf Syst Q 2015; 39(1): 245-67.
[http://dx.doi.org/10.25300/MISQ/2015/39.1.11]

[20] Alenoghena CO, Onumanyi AJ, Ohize HO, *et al.* eHealth: A survey of architectures, developments in mHealth, security concerns and solutions. Int J Environ Res Public Health 2022; 19(20): 13071.
[http://dx.doi.org/10.3390/ijerph192013071] [PMID: 36293656]

[21] Ometov A, Shubina V, Klus L, *et al.* A survey on wearable technology: History, state-of-the-art and current challenges. Comput Netw 2021; 193: 108074.
[http://dx.doi.org/10.1016/j.comnet.2021.108074]

[22] Munos B, Baker PC, Bot BM, *et al.* Mobile health: the power of wearables, sensors, and apps to

transform clinical trials. Ann N Y Acad Sci 2016; 1375(1): 3-18.
[http://dx.doi.org/10.1111/nyas.13117] [PMID: 27384501]

[23]   Bhambri P, Khang A. Managing and monitoring patient's healthcare using AI and IoT technologies In Driving Smart Medical Diagnosis Through AI-Powered Technologies and Applications. IGI Global 2024; pp. 1-23.

[24]   Haggag O, Grundy J, Abdelrazek M, Haggag S. A large scale analysis of mHealth app user reviews. Empir Softw Eng 2022; 27(7): 196.
[http://dx.doi.org/10.1007/s10664-022-10222-6] [PMID: 36246486]

[25]   Sharma A, Singh A, Verma A, Malviya R, Padarthi PK. Potential of AI in the advancement of the pharmaceutical industry. In: Pharmaceutical Industry 4.0: Future, Challenges & Application. River Publishers; 2023; pp. 107-141.

[26]   Bhatt P, Liu J, Gong Y, Wang J, Guo Y. Emerging artificial intelligence–empowered health: a scoping review. JMIR Mhealth Uhealth 2022; 10(6): e35053.
[http://dx.doi.org/10.2196/35053] [PMID: 35679107]

[27]   Al Kuwaiti A, Nazer K, Al-Reedy A, *et al.* A review of the role of artificial intelligence in healthcare. J Pers Med 2023; 13(6): 951.
[http://dx.doi.org/10.3390/jpm13060951] [PMID: 37373940]

[28]   Balakrishna S, Kumar Solanki V. A comprehensive review on AI-driven healthcare transformation. Ingenieria Solidaria 2024; 20(2): 1-30.
[http://dx.doi.org/10.16925/2357-6014.2024.02.07]

[29]   khan ZF, Alotaibi SR. Applications of artificial intelligence and big data analytics in m-health: A healthcare system perspective. J Healthc Eng 2020; 2020(1): 1-15.
[http://dx.doi.org/10.1155/2020/8894694] [PMID: 32952992]

[30]   Awad A, Trenfield SJ, Pollard TD, *et al.* Connected healthcare: Improving patient care using digital health technologies. Adv Drug Deliv Rev 2021; 178: 113958.
[http://dx.doi.org/10.1016/j.addr.2021.113958] [PMID: 34478781]

[31]   de Mattos WD, Gondim PRL. M-health solutions using 5G networks and M2M communications. IT Prof 2016; 18(3): 24-9.
[http://dx.doi.org/10.1109/MITP.2016.52]

[32]   Lamichhane B, Neupane N. Improved healthcare access in low-resource regions: A review of technological solutions arXiv preprint arXiv: 220510913 2022 2022.

[33]   Georgiou KE, Georgiou E, Satava RM. 5G use in healthcare: the future is present. JSLS. JSLS 2021; 25(4): e2021.00064.
[http://dx.doi.org/10.4293/JSLS.2021.00064]

[34]   Ahad A, Tahir M, Aman Sheikh M, Ahmed KI, Mughees A, Numani A. Technologies trend towards 5G network for smart health-care using IoT: A review. Sensors (Basel) 2020; 20(14): 4047.
[http://dx.doi.org/10.3390/s20144047] [PMID: 32708139]

[35]   Dang LM, Piran MJ, Han D, Min K, Moon H. A survey on the Internet of Things and cloud computing for healthcare. Electronics (Basel) 2019; 8(7): 768.
[http://dx.doi.org/10.3390/electronics8070768]

[36]   Jat AS, Grønli TM. Harnessing the digital revolution: a comprehensive review of mHealth applications for remote monitoring in transforming healthcare delivery. In: International Conference on Mobile Web and Intelligent Information Systems Cham: Springer 2023; 55-67.
[http://dx.doi.org/10.1007/978-3-031-39764-6_4]

[37]   Lupton D. Apps as artefacts: Towards a critical perspective on mobile health and medical apps. Societies (Basel) 2014; 4(4): 606-22.
[http://dx.doi.org/10.3390/soc4040606]

[38] George AH, Shahul A, George AS. Wearable sensors: A new way to track health and wellness. Part Uni Intl Inno J 2023; 1(4): 15-34.

[39] Shortliffe EH, Sepúlveda MJ. Clinical decision support in the era of artificial intelligence. JAMA 2018; 320(21): 2199-200.
[http://dx.doi.org/10.1001/jama.2018.17163] [PMID: 30398550]

[40] Phillips J, Babcock RA, Orbinski J. The digital response to COVID-19 : Exploring the use of digital technology for information collection, dissemination and social control in a global pandemic. J Bus Continuity Emerg Plann 2021; 14(4): 333-53.
[http://dx.doi.org/10.69554/QLQR5882] [PMID: 33962702]

[41] Assenza G, Fioravanti C, Guarino S, Petrassi V. New perspectives on wearable devices and electronic health record systems. In 2020 IEEE International Workshop on Metrology for Industry 4.0 & IoT, 2020; pp. 740-745.
[http://dx.doi.org/10.1109/MetroInd4.0IoT48571.2020.9138170]

[42] Sharma A, Verma A, Malviya R, Sekar M. Artificial-intelligence-based cloud computing techniques for patient data management. In: Artificial Intelligence for Health 4.0: Challenges and Applications. Aalborg: River Publishers 2023; p. 149-173.

[43] Cappon G, Acciaroli G, Vettoretti M, Facchinetti A, Sparacino G. Wearable continuous glucose monitoring sensors: a revolution in diabetes treatment. Electronics (Basel) 2017; 6(3): 65.
[http://dx.doi.org/10.3390/electronics6030065]

[44] Kang HS, Park HR, Kim CJ, Singh-Carlson S. Experiences of using wearable continuous glucose monitors in adults with diabetes: a qualitative descriptive study. The science of diabetes self-management and care. 2022 Oct; 48(5): 362-71.
[http://dx.doi.org/10.1177/26350106221116899]

[45] Guk K, Han G, Lim J, *et al.* Evolution of wearable devices with real-time disease monitoring for personalised healthcare. Nanomaterials (Basel) 2019; 9(6): 813.
[http://dx.doi.org/10.3390/nano9060813] [PMID: 31146479]

[46] Nandan M, Mitra S, Parai A, Jain R, Agrawal M, Singh UK. Telemedicine (e-Health, m-Health): requirements, challenges and applications. In: Bagga T, Upreti K, Kumar N, Ansari AH, Nadeem D, Eds. Designing intelligent healthcare systems, products, and services using disruptive technologies and health informatics. 1st ed. Boca Raton: CRC Press 2022; pp. 1-25.

[47] Napi NM, Zaidan AA, Zaidan BB, Albahri OS, Alsalem MA, Albahri AS. Medical emergency triage and patient prioritisation in a telemedicine environment: a systematic review. Health Technol (Berl) 2019; 9(5): 679-700.
[http://dx.doi.org/10.1007/s12553-019-00357-w]

[48] Kothamali PR, Banik S, Dandyala SS, Kumar Karne V. Advancing telemedicine and healthcare systems with AI and machine learning. Intl J Mach Learn Res Cybersec Art Intel 2024; 15(1): 177-207.

[49] El-Rashidy N, El-Sappagh S, Islam SMR, M El-Bakry H, Abdelrazek S. Mobile Health in Remote Patient Monitoring for Chronic Diseases: Principles, Trends, and Challenges. Diagnostics (Basel) 2021; 11(4): 607.

[50] Pelter MN, Quer G, Pandit J. Remote Monitoring in Cardiovascular Diseases. Curr Cardiovasc Risk Rep 2023; 17(11): 177-84.
[http://dx.doi.org/10.1007/s12170-023-00726-1]

[51] Anderson K, Burford O, Emmerton L. Mobile health apps to facilitate self-care: a qualitative study of user experiences. PLoS One 2016; 11(5): e0156164.
[http://dx.doi.org/10.1371/journal.pone.0156164] [PMID: 27214203]

[52] Filip R, Gheorghita Puscaselu R, Anchidin-Norocel L, Dimian M, Savage WK. Global challenges to public health care systems during the COVID-19 pandemic: a review of pandemic measures and

problems. J Pers Med 2022; 12(8): 1295.
[http://dx.doi.org/10.3390/jpm12081295] [PMID: 36013244]

[53] Fontelo P, Rossi E, Ackerman MJ, Marceglia S. A standards-based architecture proposal for integrating patient mHealth apps into electronic health record systems. Appl Clin Inform 2015; 6(3): 488-505.
[http://dx.doi.org/10.4338/ACI-2014-12-RA-0115] [PMID: 26448794]

[54] Alomar D, Almashmoum M, Eleftheriou I, Whelan P, Ainsworth J. The impact of patient access to electronic health records on health care engagement: systematic review. J Med Internet Res 2024; 26: e56473.
[http://dx.doi.org/10.2196/56473] [PMID: 39566058]

[55] AbuKhousa E, Mohamed N, Al-Jaroodi J. e-Health cloud: opportunities and challenges. Future Internet 2012; 4(3): 621-45.
[http://dx.doi.org/10.3390/fi4030621]

[56] Ammar N, Bailey JE, Davis RL, Shaban-Nejad A. Using a personal health library–enabled mHealth recommender system for self-management of diabetes among underserved populations: use case for knowledge graphs and linked data. JMIR Form Res 2021; 5(3): e24738.
[http://dx.doi.org/10.2196/24738] [PMID: 33724197]

[57] Oakley-Girvan I, Yunis R, Fonda SJ, *et al.* A novel smartphone application for the informal caregivers of cancer patients: Usability study. PLOS Digital Health 2023; 2(3): e0000173.
[http://dx.doi.org/10.1371/journal.pdig.0000173] [PMID: 36867639]

[58] Wang Y. Mobile appointment reminders in patient-centred care: Design and evaluation PhD dissertation Edinburg (TX). The University of Texas Rio Grande Valley 2016.

[59] Abul-Husn NS, Kenny EE. Personalised medicine and the power of electronic health records. Cell 2019; 177(1): 58-69.
[http://dx.doi.org/10.1016/j.cell.2019.02.039] [PMID: 30901549]

[60] Naseer Qureshi K, Din S, Jeon G, Piccialli F. An accurate and dynamic predictive model for a smart M-Health system using machine learning. Inf Sci 2020; 538: 486-502.
[http://dx.doi.org/10.1016/j.ins.2020.06.025]

[61] Evans D. MyFitnessPal. Br J Sports Med 2017; 51(14): 1101-2.
[http://dx.doi.org/10.1136/bjsports-2015-095538]

[62] Chong CJ, Bakry MM, Hatah E, Mohd Tahir NA, Mustafa N. Effects of mobile apps intervention on medication adherence and type 2 diabetes mellitus control: a systematic review and meta-analysis. J Telemedicine and Telecare. 2025 Mar; 31(2): 157-73. [https://doi.org/10.1177/1357633X231174933]

[63] Uscher-Pines L, Mehrotra A. Analysis of Teladoc use seems to indicate expanded access to care for patients without prior connection to a provider. Health Aff (Millwood) 2014; 33(2): 258-64.
[http://dx.doi.org/10.1377/hlthaff.2013.0989] [PMID: 24493769]

[64] Lui GY, Loughnane D, Polley C, Jayarathna T, Breen PP. The Apple Watch for monitoring mental health–related physiological symptoms: A literature review. JMIR Ment Health 2022; 9(9): e37354.
[http://dx.doi.org/10.2196/37354] [PMID: 36069848]

[65] Villarreal-Portilloa DA, Huerta-Martíneza AI, Vera-Guerreroa LS, Castro-Pastranab LI. Qualitative evaluation of the structure, content, and consistency of ten mobile applications providing drug-drug Interaction information. Lat Am J Clin Sci Med Technol 2021; 3: 106-117.

[66] Jung SY, Kim JW, Hwang H, *et al.* Development of comprehensive personal health records integrating patient-generated health data directly from Samsung S-Health and Apple Health apps: a retrospective cross-sectional observational study. JMIR Mhealth Uhealth 2019; 7(5): e12691.
[http://dx.doi.org/10.2196/12691] [PMID: 31140446]

[67] Knitza J, Mohn J, Bergmann C, *et al.* Accuracy, patient-perceived usability, and acceptance of two symptom checkers (Ada and Rheport) in rheumatology: interim results from a randomized controlled

crossover trial. Arthritis Res Ther 2021; 23(1): 112.
[http://dx.doi.org/10.1186/s13075-021-02498-8]

[68] Najjar R. Digital frontiers in healthcare: integrating mHealth, AI, and radiology for future medical diagnostics. In: Heston TF, Doarn CR, editors. A comprehensive overview of telemedicine. IntechOpen; 2024. p. 307.

[69] Verma A, Sharma A, Singh A, Malviya R, Fuloria S. Digital Assistant in the Pharmaceutical Field for Advancing Healthcare Systems. In pharmaceutical industry 4.0: Future, Challenges & Application 2023 Dec 14 (pp. 213-254). River Publishers.

[70] Nasi G, Cucciniello M, Guerrazzi C. The performance of mHealth in cancer supportive care: a research agenda. J Med Internet Res 2015; 17(1): e9.
[http://dx.doi.org/10.2196/jmir.3764] [PMID: 25720295]

[71] Hernandez Silva E, Lawler S, Langbecker D. The effectiveness of mHealth for self-management in improving pain, psychological distress, fatigue, and sleep in cancer survivors: a systematic review. J Cancer Surviv 2019; 13(1): 97-107.
[http://dx.doi.org/10.1007/s11764-018-0730-8] [PMID: 30635865]

[72] Tsang KCH, Pinnock H, Wilson AM, Shah SA. Application of machine learning algorithms for asthma management with mHealth: a clinical review. J Asthma Allergy 2022; 15: 855-73.
[http://dx.doi.org/10.2147/JAA.S285742] [PMID: 35791395]

[73] Khusial RJ, Honkoop PJ, Usmani O, *et al.* Effectiveness of myAirCoach: a mHealth self-management system in asthma. J Allergy Clin Immunol Pract 2020; 8(6): 1972-1979.e8.
[http://dx.doi.org/10.1016/j.jaip.2020.02.018] [PMID: 32142961]

[74] Yotsu RR, Itoh S, Yao KA, *et al.* The early detection and case management of skin diseases with a mHealth App (eSkinHealth): protocol for a mixed methods pilot study in Cote d'Ivoire. JMIR Res Protoc 2022; 11(9): e39867.
[http://dx.doi.org/10.2196/39867] [PMID: 35922062]

[75] Kvedarienė V, Burzdikaitė P, Česnavičiūtė I. mHealth and telemedicine utility in the monitoring of allergic diseases. Front Allergy 2022; 3: 919746.

[76] Madhvapathy SR, Wang H, Kong J, *et al.* Reliable, low-cost, fully integrated hydration sensors for monitoring and diagnosis of inflammatory skin diseases in any environment. Sci Adv 2020; 6(49): eabd7146.
[http://dx.doi.org/10.1126/sciadv.abd7146] [PMID: 33277260]

[77] Buneviciene I, Mekary RA, Smith TR, Onnela JP, Bunevicius A. Can mHealth interventions improve the quality of life of cancer patients? A systematic review and meta-analysis. Critical reviews in oncology/haematology. 2021 Jan 1; 157:103123.

[78] Farzandipour M, Nabovati E, Sharif R, Arani M, Anvari S. Patient self-management of asthma using mobile health applications: a systematic review of the functionalities and effects. Appl Clin Inform 2017; 8(4): 1068-81.
[http://dx.doi.org/10.4338/ACI-2017-07-R-0116] [PMID: 29241254]

[79] Yotsu RR, Almamy D, Vagamon B, *et al.* A mHealth app (skin health) for detecting and managing skin diseases in resource-limited settings: mixed methods pilot study. JMIR Dermatology 2023; 6: e46295.
[http://dx.doi.org/10.2196/46295] [PMID: 37632977]

[80] Marzano L, Bardill A, Fields B, *et al.* The application of mHealth to mental health: opportunities and challenges. Lancet Psychiatry 2015; 2(10): 942-8.
[http://dx.doi.org/10.1016/S2215-0366(15)00268-0] [PMID: 26462228]

[81] Price M, Yuen EK, Goetter EM, *et al.* mHealth: a mechanism to deliver more accessible, more effective mental health care. Clin Psychol Psychother 2014; 21(5): 427-36.
[http://dx.doi.org/10.1002/cpp.1855] [PMID: 23918764]

[82]   Bidargaddi N, Schrader G, Klasnja P, Licinio J, Murphy S. Designing m-Health interventions for precision mental health support. Transl Psychiatry 2020; 10(1): 222.
[http://dx.doi.org/10.1038/s41398-020-00895-2] [PMID: 32636358]

[83]   Chan S, Li L, Torous J, Gratzer D, Yellowlees PM. Review and implementation of self-help and automated tools in mental health care. Psychiatr Clin North Am 2019; 42(4): 597-609.
[http://dx.doi.org/10.1016/j.psc.2019.07.001] [PMID: 31672210]

[84]   Rivera-Romero O, Gabarron E, Ropero J, Denecke K. Designing personalised mHealth solutions: An overview. J Biomed Inform 2023; 146: 104500.
[http://dx.doi.org/10.1016/j.jbi.2023.104500] [PMID: 37722446]

[85]   Gan DZQ, McGillivray L, Larsen ME, Christensen H, Torok M. Technology-supported strategies for promoting user engagement with digital mental health interventions: A systematic review. Digit Health 2022; 8
[http://dx.doi.org/10.1177/20552076221098268] [PMID: 35677785]

[86]   Chen H, Chai Y, Dong L, Niu W, Zhang P. Effectiveness and appropriateness of mHealth interventions for maternal and child health: systematic review. JMIR Mhealth Uhealth 2018; 6(1): e7.
[http://dx.doi.org/10.2196/mhealth.8998] [PMID: 29317380]

[87]   Lee SH, Nurmatov UB, Nwaru BI, Mukherjee M, Grant L, Pagliari C. Effectiveness of mHealth interventions for maternal, newborn and child health in low– and middle–income countries: Systematic review and meta–analysis. J Glob Health 2016; 6(1): 010401.
[http://dx.doi.org/10.7189/jogh.06.010401] [PMID: 26649177]

[88]   Gilano G, Dekker A, Fijten R. The role of mHealth intervention to improve maternal and child health: A provider-based qualitative study in Southern Ethiopia. PLoS One 2024; 19(2): e0295539.
[http://dx.doi.org/10.1371/journal.pone.0295539] [PMID: 38329947]

[89]   Virani A, Duffett-Leger L, Letourneau N. Parents' use of mobile applications in the first year of parenthood: a narrative review of the literature. Health Technol (Berl) 2021; 5: 1-20.

[90]   Rimmer JH, Wilroy J, Galea P, Jeter A, Lai BW. Retrospective evaluation of a pilot eHealth/mHealth telewellness program for people with disabilities: Mindfulness, Exercise, and Nutrition To Optimize Resilience (MENTOR). mHealth 2022; 8: 15.
[http://dx.doi.org/10.21037/mhealth-21-34] [PMID: 35449508]

[91]   Chuckun V, Coonjan G, Nagowah L. Enabling the Disabled using mHealth. In: 2019 Conference on Next Generation Computing Applications (NextComp) 2019; 1-6.

[92]   Frisby C, Eikelboom R, Mahomed-Asmail F, Kuper H, Swanepoel DW. M-Health applications for hearing loss: a scoping review. Telemed J E Health 2022; 28(8): 1090-9.
[http://dx.doi.org/10.1089/tmj.2021.0460] [PMID: 34967683]

[93]   Nandan M, Mitra S, Parai A, Jain R, Agrawal M, Singh UK. Telemedicine (e-Health, m-Health): requirements, challenges and applications. In: Bagga T, Upreti K, Kumar N, Ansari AH, Nadeem D, Eds. Designing intelligent healthcare systems, products, and services using disruptive technologies and health informatics. 1st ed. Boca Raton: CRC Press 2022; pp. 1-25.

[94]   Pickard Strange M, Booth A, Akiki M, Wieringa S, Shaw SE. The role of virtual consulting in developing environmentally sustainable health care: a systematic literature review. J Med Internet Res 2023; 25: e44823.
[http://dx.doi.org/10.2196/44823] [PMID: 37133914]

[95]   Iribarren SJ, Cato K, Falzon L, Stone PW. What is the economic evidence for mHealth? A systematic review of economic evaluations of mHealth solutions. PLoS One 2017; 12(2): e0170581.
[http://dx.doi.org/10.1371/journal.pone.0170581] [PMID: 28152012]

[96]   Damar M, Kop O, Şaylan ÖF, Özen A, Çakmak ÜE, Erenay FS. Digital Health: the critical value of mobile technology for the health sector, different application examples from the world and current trends. J Emer Comp Techn 2024 Dec; 4(1): 25-37.

[http://dx.doi.org/10.57020/ject.1514154]

[97] Aminabee S. The future of healthcare and patient-centric care: Digital innovations, trends, and predictions In: Emerging Technologies for Health Literacy and Medical Practice. IGI Global 2024; pp. 240-62.
[http://dx.doi.org/10.4018/979-8-3693-1214-8.ch012]

[98] Boulos MN, Brewer AC, Karimkhani C, Buller DB, Dellavalle RP. Mobile medical and health apps: state of the art, concerns, regulatory control and certification. Online J Public Health Inform 2014; 5(3): 229.
[PMID: 24683442]

[99] Kao CK, Liebovitz DM. Consumer mobile health apps: current state, barriers, and future directions. PM R 2017; 9(5S): S106-15.
[http://dx.doi.org/10.1016/j.pmrj.2017.02.018] [PMID: 28527495]

[100] Prasad S. Designing for scalability and trustworthiness in health systems. In: Distributed Computing and Internet Technology: 11th International Conference, ICDCIT 2015, Bhubaneswar, India, Cham: Springer International Publishing 2015; pp. 114-3.

[101] Niekrenz L, Spreckelsen C. How to design effective educational videos for teaching evidence-based medicine to undergraduate learners–systematic review with complementing qualitative research to develop a practicable guide. Medical education online 2024 Dec 31; 29(1): 2339569.
[https://doi.org/10.1080/10872981.2024.2339569]

[102] Kim H, Goldsmith JV, Sengupta S, *et al.* Mobile health application and e-health literacy: opportunities and concerns for cancer patients and caregivers. J Cancer Educ 2019; 34(1): 3-8.
[http://dx.doi.org/10.1007/s13187-017-1293-5] [PMID: 29139070]

[103] Kruse C, Betancourt J, Ortiz S, Valdes Luna SM, Bamrah IK, Segovia N. Barriers to the use of mobile health in improving health outcomes in developing countries: systematic review. J Med Internet Res 2019; 21(10): e13263.
[http://dx.doi.org/10.2196/13263] [PMID: 31593543]

[104] Martínez-Pérez B, de la Torre-Díez I, López-Coronado M. Privacy and security in mobile health apps: a review and recommendations. J Med Syst 2015; 39(1): 181.
[http://dx.doi.org/10.1007/s10916-014-0181-3] [PMID: 25486895]

[105] Hampshire K, Mwase-Vuma T, Alemu K, *et al.* Informal mhealth at scale in Africa: Opportunities and challenges. World Dev 2021; 140: 105257.
[http://dx.doi.org/10.1016/j.worlddev.2020.105257] [PMID: 33814676]

[106] Källander K, Tibenderana JK, Akpogheneta OJ, *et al.* Mobile health (mHealth) approaches and lessons for increased performance and retention of community health workers in low- and middle-income countries: a review. J Med Internet Res 2013; 15(1): e17.
[http://dx.doi.org/10.2196/jmir.2130] [PMID: 23353680]

CHAPTER 2

Optimising Hospital Management Systems

Zeba Siddiqui[1], Ashish Verma[2], Akanksha Sharma[3], Shaweta Sharma[4], Sunita[3] and Akhil Sharma[3],*

[1] *Amity Institute of Pharmacy, Amity University, Gwalior, Madhya Pradesh 474005, India*

[2] *Mangalmay Pharmacy College, Greater Noida, Uttar Pradesh 201306, India*

[3] *R.J. College of Pharmacy, Raipur, Gharbara, Tappal, Khair, Uttar Pradesh 202165, India*

[4] *School of Medical and Allied Sciences, Galgotias University, Yamuna Expressway, Gautam Buddha Nagar, Uttar Pradesh 201310, India*

Abstract: Hospital Management Systems (HMS) play an important role in improving the quality and effectiveness of healthcare provision by handling patient information, inventory, staff, and finances. However, current challenges, such as data fragmentation, resource allocation inefficiencies, and administrative burdens, hinder their optimal functioning. Optimising HMS is essential for addressing these issues and ensuring seamless healthcare operations. This chapter explores the key features of HMS, including patient info management, inventory management, staff management, and finance systems. It further explores the technology driving optimisation, including Artificial Intelligence (AI) for predictive analytics and scheduling, Blockchain for secure data management, Internet of Things (IoT) for real-time monitoring, and Cloud computing for scalable data storage and remote access. The chapter discusses automation and workflow optimisation techniques that eliminate manual processes and streamline interfacing between departments. It also underscores system integration, interoperability and compliance with regulations in health care. The chapter concluded by discussing some future trends in HMS, where robotics is set to play a crucial role, and the future of HMS with emerging technologies such as 5G and edge computing. By leveraging these innovations, healthcare facilities can enhance service delivery, decrease operational costs, and improve patient care.

Keywords: Artificial intelligence, Automation, Blockchain, Cloud computing, IoT, Hospital management systems, Interoperability, Optimisation.

---

* **Corresponding author Akhil Sharma:** R.J. College of Pharmacy, Raipur, Gharbara, Tappal, Khair, Uttar Pradesh 202165, India; E-mail: xs2akhil@gmail.com

Akhil Sharma, Shaweta Sharma, Pankaj Kumar Singh & Neeraj Kumar Fuloria (Eds.)

INTRODUCTION

Hospital Management Systems (HMS) are well-integrated systems to manage the standard hospital functions. Such systems cover a wide range of functions, such as patient registration, appointments, medical records, billing, inventory, and reporting. HMS uses state-of-the-art technology to digitise and unify administrative, clinical, and financial processes, ensuring integrated communication between departments. HMS simplifies decision-making and streamlines operational efficiency by offering real-time access to critical data. These systems usually consist of modular components, enabling a healthcare provider to use solutions based on the identified needs. The implementation of HMS is vital in modern healthcare environments, as it minimises mistakes, optimises resources, and improves patient satisfaction while also complying with regulatory standards [1 - 3].

Current Challenges in Traditional HMS

Traditional Hospital Management Systems (HMS) face several challenges that hinder their ability to meet the demands of modern healthcare delivery. One of the primary issues is the reliance on outdated, siloed systems that lack interoperability. Such systems typically block seamless interdepartmental communication, resulting in fragmented care delivery and redundancies. For example, if patient data are recorded in different databases, then comprehensive patient data profiling may demand manual integration, leading to potential errors in treatment and delays [4].

The scalability of traditional HMS is another critical issue. These systems tend to offer limited capabilities when health systems grow, resulting in increased data volumes and more users. This results in system failures, damaging performance in high-critical time frames. Additionally, many traditional systems lack advanced analytics capabilities, hindering the ability to derive actionable insights from data for decision-making [5].

Cybersecurity poses a pressing issue for conventional healthcare management systems as well, since antiquated security protocols frequently leave these platforms vulnerable to intrusions. Sensitive patient details risk exposure to unauthorised access through deficient encryption and authentication mechanisms, priming regulatory noncompliance and reputational damage. Furthermore, conventional systems frequently present arduous learning curves for users owing to their unsuitability for human operators, inducing reluctance toward adoption among medical personnel. Cost remains a barrier, particularly for smaller and mid-sized medical facilities [6 - 8].

Traditional solutions regularly involve prohibitive upfront costs, including licensing, hardware expenses, and maintenance fees. These fiscal constraints preclude widespread implementation, especially in resource-constrained settings. Finally, the lack of integration with emerging technologies, such as the Internet of Things, artificial intelligence, and blockchain, circumscribes the potential of conventional healthcare management systems to propel medical progress and enhance patient care. Addressing these challenges is paramount to transitioning toward optimised next-generation solutions with the elasticity to meet evolving healthcare needs [9, 10].

Importance of Optimization in Healthcare Delivery

With the soaring demand for efficient and effective medical services growing in an increasingly complex environment, healthcare delivery has become one of those domains where optimisation has become a necessity. The healthcare sector is under pressure from increased demand and reduced capacity, rising costs and an increasingly ageing population. Optimisation is about using technology, data analytics and process reengineering to utilise resources in the best possible way, maximise the outcomes for each patient, and minimise waste. It expedites care delivery by optimising workflows, minimising patient wait times, and avoiding duplications in efforts [11, 12].

Optimised healthcare delivery fosters the improved delivery of care and translates into better patient experiences with quicker access to healthcare and personalised care. It also improves the efficiency of hospitals' operations by automating recurring jobs, thus allowing healthcare professionals to devote more time to patients. In addition, it also aids in financial sustainability by managing the cost and optimising the revenue cycles. By leveraging predictive analytics as well as AI-driven tools, organisations will predict patient needs, manage resources to deliver services to patients and equitably deliver services [13, 14].

Moreover, optimisation is critical for solving health equity. Telemedicine and Mobile Health Solutions enable healthcare providers to extend services to remote and underserved areas. It further stimulates innovation and the use of advanced medical devices, technology and treatments. Ultimately, optimisation will help reform these healthcare systems into more patient-centred, resilient, and responsive frameworks [15].

FEATURES OF OPTIMIZED HOSPITAL MANAGEMENT SYSTEMS (HMS)

Optimised Hospital management systems (HMS) are crucial in effective healthcare delivery and infusing technology into operations. Patient information management makes health records accurate and accessible [16]. Healthcare inventory and supply chain management help to ensure that medical supplies are tracked and processed accurately for procurement across various healthcare facilities. Staff management improves the efficiency of the workforce through automated scheduling and performance tracking. While, financial management deals with proper invoicing and insurance claims processing. Altogether, this helps to optimise the entire process, which leads to better patient care, operational cost savings, and overall hospital efficiency through standardised processes, data-driven decisions, and transparency [17 - 19]. The various features of optimised hospital management systems are depicted in Fig. (**1**).

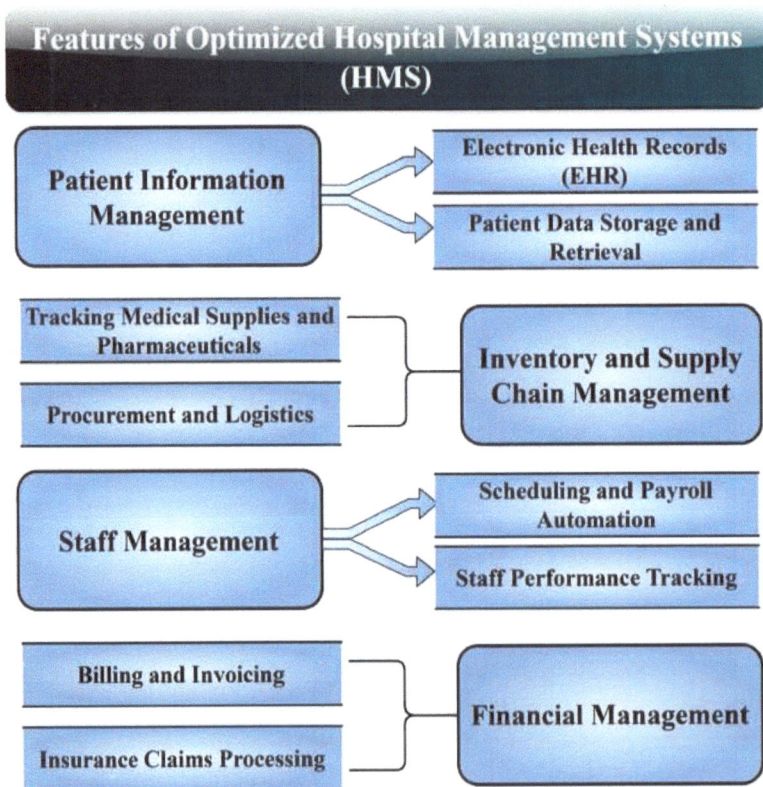

Fig. (1). Features of optimized hospital management systems.

Patient Information Management

Patient information management is the process in which accurate records or data about patients are collected, stored, processed, and made available accordingly. It includes demographic information, medical history, allergies, and treatment plans so that all stakeholders have updated information. EHR Integration streamlines workflows, lessens testing redundancy, and enhances coordination. With easy-to-use interfaces, healthcare providers benefit from having real-time access to patient information that everyone involved in the care can have readily available to them. Features such as strong encryption and access controls protect data from unauthorised access and keep it compliant with regulatory standards. Management of information about patients improves the quality of care and availability of patient outcomes and facilitates the efficient functioning of the hospital [20 - 22].

Electronic Health Records (EHR)

EHRs (electronic health records) are digital copies of patients' medical histories that make it easier for health providers to access and store data. Electronic health records (EHRs) are secure, real-time digital patient records with a patient data summary that may include a patient's medical history, diagnoses, treatment plans, immunisation records, and test results, enabling smooth communication between providers, improving care coordination, ensuring proper medical assistance, and eliminating medical mistakes. By yielding past treatments and subsequent outcomes, EHRs support decisions grounded in evidence. Integration with diagnostic tools and wearables extends the possibility of real-time data collection, thereby facilitating proactive care. Population health is supported through advanced features such as data analytics and predictive modelling [23, 24].

Patient Data Storage and Retrieval

Efficient patient data storage and retrieval are critical in modern healthcare settings. Advanced database systems ensure secure, scalable storage of vast amounts of patient data. Cloud solutions provide flexibility, allowing authorised personnel to access data anytime and anywhere while minimising infrastructure expenditure [25]. Sensitive data, including personally identifiable information, is kept safe from breaches using encryption, multi-factor authentication, and role-based access controls. Search algorithms and metadata tagging of records have created efficient retrieval systems of specific patient medical information in healthcare. This integration enables continuous and seamless sharing of data between departments by integrating with EHR and other hospital systems. Utilities faced with multi-hospital consolidated data analysis, optimisation, and planning projects can even use ready-made solutions and overcome organisational siloes by systematically addressing clinical decision-making, operational efficiency, and patient satisfaction [26, 27].

Inventory and Supply Chain Management

Inventory and supply chain management are key to the uninterrupted functioning of a hospital. Tracking medical supplies, equipment, and pharmaceuticals effectively prevents patient care from being hindered due to supply stock-outs, overstocking, and waste. The primary purpose of the HMS is to track inventory in real-time so that hospital administrators have an up-to-the-moment view of stock levels in all hospital departments. Automated alerts can notify when supplies are running low or when products approach their expiration dates. This ensures that essential supplies are always available, thereby avoiding delays in treatment. Moreover, integrating inventory management with procurement processes streamlines order fulfilment, enhancing overall efficiency [28, 29].

Tracking Medical Supplies and Pharmaceuticals

The key element of hospital management systems is the tracking of medical supplies and pharmaceuticals. Hospitals have enormous volumes of prescriptions, surgical instruments, and medical devices in constant circulation, which necessitates the use of real-time monitoring methods to avoid scarcity and minimise mistakes [30]. HMS delivers centralised databases to record inventory information by numbers, usage rates, due dates, and lot numbers. The RFID tracking systems are combined with barcode scanning systems, allowing the movement of stock to be accurately tracked. Such tools aid in traceability and keep track of compliance with regulations. Additionally, the data collected provides hospitals with data on usage trends, ensuring that they can predict and plan for future demand in advance. In addition to accurate tracking supporting better management of resequencing, it is critical to ensure patient safety by avoiding administering expired or the wrong medications. This tracking provides crucial benefits such as reduced waste, better efficiency in the operation process, and optimised stock replenishment where patient care is involved [31 - 33].

Procurement and Logistics

Hospital supply chain functions in procurement and logistics are critical for ensuring the uninterrupted flow of medical supplies and pharmaceuticals. The procurement process includes obtaining premium quality products from trustworthy suppliers at reasonable prices. An HMS solution that has been optimised will be able to help reduce procurement bottlenecks by automating orders, tracking vendor performance, and ensuring compliance with contracts and regulatory requirements [34]. Logistics plays a significant role in maintaining timely patient service, and an efficiently integrated system delivers timely and reduced waiting time for patient care. Predictive analytics can tackle demand variability challenges, as hospitals have largely predictable utilisation patterns based on historical data. In addition, a solid logistics network arranges the transportation and storage of goods, handling stock at different areas of the hospital, from wards to working theatres to drug stores. The global pandemic has highlighted that automated reorder systems can reduce errors and ensure that critical inventories are indeed available for use [35, 36].

Staff Management

Staff management is an integral part of the optimum hospital management system (HMS) for the workflow to function smoothly. It includes hiring, training, assigning healthcare staff, and dealing with work schedules and leave requests. A well-organized staff management module ensures that the hospital has the right staff at the right time, which leads to a better quality of care delivery and helps improve key operational efficiencies. Within the system, administrators can track staff availability, address schedule conflicts, and confirm that no department is overworked or understaffed. Simplified staff management leads to fewer operational inefficiencies and enables the facility to provide quality care [37, 38].

Scheduling and Payroll Automation

The applications of scheduling and payroll automation *via* an HMS ensure there are minimal manual errors, operational efficiency, and timely payment. Automated scheduling, instead of manual scheduling, automates shift assignments based on staff availability and certifications to help support workload requirements while meeting patient care needs. The use of sophisticated algorithms will optimise the process of scheduling staff, therefore decreasing scheduling conflicts and facilitating better satisfaction [39].

HMS ensure accurate payroll calculations due to automatic integration with attendance and work hours tracking for payroll automation. Such a system automates the payroll processing of salaries, bonuses, and other benefits to ensure that they are calculated and delivered on time, minimising the potential for human errors or fraud [40]. Time-tracking devices like biometric scanners or employee mobile app integrations enable easy data capture for payroll processing. Additionally, the system can manage varying payment structures for different staff categories, such as doctors, nurses, and administrative personnel, ensuring compliance with labour laws and internal policies. Combining this approach into one process provides not only a reduction in time taken but also an amplification of transparency, creating trust, reducing administrative burden, and operational efficiencies. Automation of scheduling and payroll allows hospitals to invest their time and energy into patient care while still keeping staff happy and ensuring operational integrity [41, 42].

Staff Performance Tracking

An integral feature of an optimised HMS is staff performance tracking, which is aimed at tracking the speedy day-to-day operations of the healthcare staff. It leverages data-driven insights to assess individual and team performance against defined key performance indicators. It implements data on metrics like patient feedback, visit completion, time management, and clinical outcomes. This enables administrators to pinpoint where staff excel and where additional training or support may be needed. This allows hospitals to create a culture of ongoing learning, set goals for professional development, and give specialised feedback to staff based on performance data [43, 44].

Performance tracking helps identify high-performing individuals who can be rewarded or promoted while also highlighting underperforming staff who may require additional resources or interventions. Conducting performance evaluations regularly helps ensure that the members of staff stay engaged, motivated, and aligned with the hospital's targets, consequently enhancing the efficiency of patient care services and the hospital's overall operations. It can improve collaboration amongst team members and resolve systemic problems using performance data. The transparency brought about by performance feedback enables hospitals to design customised training programs to fill skill gaps and build workforce capacities. This model creates a healthcare ecosystem that is inherently more dynamic, responsive, and patient-centred [45, 46].

Financial Management

Hospital financial management has various perspectives, such as monitoring, controlling, and optimising financial activities through multiple stages at the hospital's external and internal levels to ensure a sustainable level of operations. Essential elements are budget management, revenue generation, and cost-control tools. A definite bottleneck that HMS can tackle will enable the real-time traceability of cash transactions, proper reporting, and compliance with financial regulations. This allows the effective management of expenses, billing processes, and revenue collection through the use of specialised financial management software in sub-systems. Financial workflows can be streamlined, enabling hospitals to save on operational costs, ensuring timely payments and improving cash flow. A well-configured HMS can also assist in predictive analytics for budget forecasting, which leads to improved decision-making and better resource allocation [47, 48].

Billing and Invoicing

Billing and invoicing are the most fundamental processes of hospital management. A well-designed HMS automatically generates invoices for services rendered against the patient, helping ensure correctness and conformity. It integrates with EHR systems to extract data such as patient demographics, treatment codes, and cost details, reducing the chance of human error. It helps streamline the whole billing cycle from generating the first invoice to dispatching it to the insurance companies or patients and tracking payment status in real-time [49].

A high-level HMS can also handle different billing forms, like direct patient billing and insurance claims processing. Quick and easy automated invoice generation reduces the need for manual data entry, speeds up the billing process, and improves cash flow through the acceleration of payment cycles. It allows billing discrepancies to be detected early, which helps avoid revenue losses and improves financial health. Additionally, a well-optimized HMS makes billing data easily accessible when it comes to financial reporting, which supports audits and compliance with regulations [50].

Insurance Claims Processing

Processing insurance claims is one of the most involved yet crucial functions in hospital management. A well-optimized HMS streamlines this process further through the automation of some critical functions like submissions, tracking and reconciliations of claims to simplify the claims processing. The system electronically submits claims to insurance carriers, which minimises the possibility of errors experienced during manual submission [51]. It complies with industry standards and helps track the claim's status in real-time. HMS is capable of being interfaced with verification systems used by insurance providers, allowing the HMS to check with the appropriate health insurance system for a specific patient to find coverage information far more seamlessly when pre-authorization is necessary [52].

This helps minimise claim denials, ensuring that only valid claims get processed. The system also allows payment status tracking and can produce extensive reports on average claim processing times and results. An optimised HMS automates these tasks to minimise administrative workload on staff while reducing the risk of claim errors and adding to the overall operational efficiency. This will not only enhance the cash flow of the hospital but also prevent under-reporting and over-expenditure of patients during admission and discharge, thereby improving its financial records and insurance compliance [53].

TECHNOLOGIES FOR OPTIMIZING HOSPITAL MANAGEMENT

With the development of technology, the management of hospitals is different, reaching high-level operational efficiency and providing better patient care. AI, Blockchain, IoT, and Cloud Computing have their unique importance in reducing friction in hospital operations, predicting demand for patients, ensuring data security, and facilitating correct communication. These technologies play a key role not just in assisting clinical functions but also in managing administrative functions, optimising resource utilisation, and reducing operational costs [54]. Technologies used in optimising hospital management systems are summarised in Fig. (**2**).

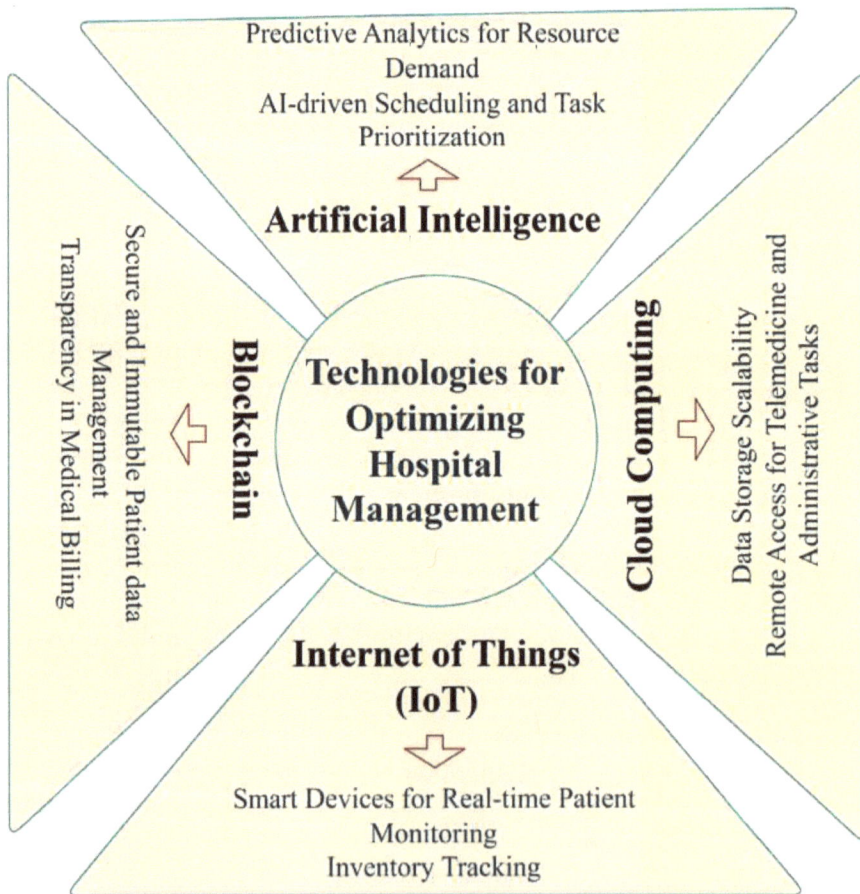

Fig. (2). Technologies for optimizing hospital management systems.

Artificial Intelligence (AI) in Hospital Management

Hospital management is changing now with Artificial Intelligence (AI), automating and optimising all administrative and clinical responsibilities. With the ability to analyse large volumes of data, AI systems contribute to timely decision-making, the minimisation of human error, and better healthcare. AI can improve the efficiency of hospitals and the satisfaction of patients through the use of machine learning algorithms and predictive models that predict outcomes, optimise staff allocation, and enhance operational workflows within the healthcare systems [55].

Predictive Analytics for Resource Demand

AI-driven predictive analytics are changing the way hospitals plan for and utilise their resources, helping them predict demand for medical resources like beds, staff, and equipment. With predictive models that can analyse historical data, patient admission patterns, and external factors such as a pandemic, hospitals can predict peak demand periods and prepare to help humans prepare for intervention-related needs [56]. For example, AI can predict surges in patient volume during flu seasons or emergencies, allowing hospitals to adjust staffing levels and prepare necessary supplies in advance proactively. Taking this proactive stance can help to mitigate the bottlenecks, lower the waiting periods, and guarantee that essential resources will be ready when needed the most. In addition, predictive analytics can also help figure out how many ICU beds to be used based on the trend of the patient severity levels or predict equipment failures, timely maintenance, minimise downtime, *etc*. Using predictive models, hospitals can establish multi-channel data-driven demand management strategies, yielding improvement in operational efficiency and patient care outcomes [57, 58].

AI-driven Scheduling and Task Prioritization

Another hospital management innovation is AI-driven scheduling and task prioritisation. AI can automate healthcare professionals' scheduling by optimising shifts based on patient volume, staff expertise, and operational needs. AI then uses machine learning algorithms to analyse the historical patient admission data and treatment durations for all different types of patients to predict and adjust the schedules to meet peak times best. AI systems, for example, can suggest more staff during busy hours or reshuffle bookings to ensure that the patient flow will be in its most optimal condition [59].

For task prioritisation, AI helps assess the urgency of various medical duties and aids in workflow management by ensuring that the most critical tasks are performed first. This minimises bottlenecks, facilitates faster response times, and maximises the quality of patient care. Moreover, AI tools can assist in prioritising administrative tasks, such as billing and documentation, ensuring that non-clinical duties do not overwhelm healthcare providers. By integrating AI into scheduling and task prioritisation, hospitals can enhance both operational efficiency and the quality of patient care [60].

Blockchain in Hospital Management

Blockchain technology is a potential game-changer for hospital management in terms of secure, transparent, effective and efficient management of patient data, medical billing, and supply chain management. Blockchain has the potential to replace conventional vulnerabilities by utilising decentralised, immutable ledgers, making it a strong candidate for maintaining sensitive data. This increase augments the privacy of the data, builds confidence, and diminishes business mistakes. With the smooth management of operations, from record-keeping of patients to securing transactions from unauthorised access, blockchain is used in the hospital management system [61].

Secure and Immutable Patient Data Management

The capacity of blockchain to keep track of and safeguard patient data is among the significant benefits it provides for the healthcare industry. Conventional electronic health record (EHR) systems based on centralised databases mean that the same cyberattacks can target clinical data as computers and must be defended against wholesale unauthorised access. Blockchain tackles this problem with a distributed ledger that guarantees that patient data remains encrypted and can never be changed or removed once any information is entered [62].

It provides an audit trail that helps rarely auditable records for patients and makes it immensely unfeasible for malware or unauthorised parties to tamper with data. Blockchain also allows data to be shared among various healthcare providers without any risk to patient data, enabling patients to control their information better. With this distribution mechanism, both patients can access their medical records anywhere at any time, and institutions can view and update them securely [63].

Blockchain also reduces administrative overhead by automating processes like patient consent management, streamlining workflows, and ensuring accurate documentation. This enables hospitals to improve the accuracy and efficiency of data while reducing data management costs and fraud prevention [64].

Transparency in Medical Billing

By making records of all transactions transparent, traceable, and incorruptible, blockchain could serve a key role in helping to optimise the medical billing process. Medical billing in conventional hospital management systems is usually subject to error, fraud, and discrepancies, which in turn cause problems such as overcharging or mismanagement of insurance claims. Blockchain solves this problem by building permanent logs for every medical service performed [65].

For example, each billable encounter, such as consultation, treatment or procedure, is recorded on a distributed ledger, and the patient and the healthcare provider can check whether the charge is valid and correct. This adds transparency, reduces billing disputes, and improves accountability by only billing patients for services actually provided. Moreover, due to the transparency of insurance on the blockchain, it is easier to process an insurance claim as the record of the services rendered is straightforward and can be audited quickly [66].

This helps improve trust in the hospital or patient insurance companies, as blockchain has reduced the administrative costs associated with fraud. Blockchain using smart contracts can automatically handle billing, which guarantees compliance with insurance policies and further optimises the hospital revenue cycle process. In the end, these types of technology result in a streamlined medical billing process based on efficiency, accuracy, and transparency, which benefits the myriad stakeholders involved [67].

Internet of Things (IoT) in Hospital Management

The IoT is an important technology that will change the way hospitals are managed through devices that communicate with each other to exchange data in real time. This can help hospitals increase operational capabilities, deliver better care, and save costs using IoT. Wearables, sensors, and RFID tags are smart healthcare devices that keep patient health in check and are used for equipment tracking and asset management. The use of IoT-based systems guarantees proper inventory management, medical device tracking, and data-driven decision-making. IoT technology automates and optimises processes, improving the management of workflow, patient safety, and the general efficiency of the hospital [68].

Smart Devices for Management

Smart devices that use the IoT have revolutionised hospital management, offering benefits that go from patient experience to operational efficiency. Hospitals can assimilate smart medical devices like health monitors, automated medication dispensers, smart infusion pumps, and real-time location services (RTLS) into their management system to promote the clinical and administrative components of healthcare [69].

Wearable Health Monitors

The devices monitor vital parameters like heart rate, blood pressure, and oxygen levels and transmit data straight away to healthcare providers. It enables continuous monitoring of the patients, which eliminates the need for frequent physical checks and allows for timely intervention. Wearables afford rich data that can also be mined for health trends, advance the prediction of complications, and better outcomes [70].

Automated Medication Dispensers

With the help of IoT-powered dispensers, medication schedules and dosages are monitored, minimising human errors. These devices send alerts to staff if there are discrepancies or missed doses by integrating with hospital databases and creating an audit trail for compliance. It improves patient safety and makes computer-assisted medication management much more efficient [71].

Smart Infusion Pumps

It controls intravenous drug delivery with remarkable accuracy. More specifically, IoT infusion pumps will communicate with a central monitoring system at the hospital for real-time monitoring of medications administered. These notifications may also be transmitted directly to health professionals who provide better management and lower risks in case of failures, alerts to patients, or deviated doses [72].

Real-Time Location Services (RTLS)

RTLS technology identifies RFID tags that are put on hospital assets, including medical equipment, wheelchairs, and IV pumps. When there are no manual tracking methods, hospitals will have a constant monitoring solution in hand to ensure that relevant equipment and assets are fully functional and readily available when required. Moreover, RTLS allows staff to locate and retrieve equipment in a matter of seconds, thereby reducing searching time and enhancing workflow efficiency [73].

Environmental Monitoring

IoT sensors are deployed to monitor the external environmental factors in critical areas such as the operating rooms and drug storage area with sensors that can monitor parameters such as temperature, humidity, and air quality. The sensors guarantee compliance with safety standards and help to maintain optimal environmental conditions for patient care, medication storage, and equipment functionality [74].

Cloud Computing in Hospital Management

Cloud technology has emerged as a game-changer, bringing new cloud-based solutions and services that enhance hospital management. This will enable cross-departmental data storage, resource management, and collaboration. Cloud services help hospitals reduce management, real-time sharing of patient data, and overall administration time. Cloud-based software is able to integrate many functions, such as Electronic Health Records (EHR), patient scheduling, and billing, to offer a unified and accessible system for healthcare providers and patients alike [75].

Data Storage Scalability

Cloud computing provides unmatched scalability to hospitals, which is a key advantage when it comes to storing volumes of healthcare data that are growing exponentially. Traditional on-premise storage systems are often limited due to a lack of physical space and the ability to respond quickly to ever-growing data needs. On the other hand, cloud platforms offer effectively infinite storage, giving hospitals the opportunity to store considerable amounts of patient data, imaging files, and medical records safely. Hospitals can scale their storage when needed without the need to purchase expensive new hardware. Therefore, it is cost-effective for both large and small institutions [76].

Cloud storage is flexible enough for hospitals to deploy solid backup and disaster recovery plans, keeping the data safe from any loss from technical faults or natural disasters. Besides, hospitals can rapidly scale up their storage resources during peak demand months, when both data volume and demand increase, especially during pandemics, for instance. The on-demand nature of cloud storage allows patients to pay only for the amount of storage they are actually using, maximising cost savings while still allowing them to manage a spike in data burdens. In addition, cloud storage solutions often have automated data management tools, increasing efficacy by policy-based data classification, retrieval, and access [77].

Remote Access for Telemedicine and Administrative Tasks

The use of cloud computing also significantly improves remote access to a hospital management system, which is one of the key features that have great significance in telemedicine and administrative functionalities. Telemedicine is a crucial modern healthcare service that is adding significant importance, especially for patients in rural or underserved regions with little to no access to healthcare facilities. The cloud assists doctors in providing remote consultations, remote monitoring of patient health and status, and accessing real-time electronic patient records, resulting in uninterrupted care to patients, especially in times of crisis [78].

Cloud computing enables hospital staff to manage scheduling, billing, patient intake, and more from anywhere, an essential factor for administrative functions when hybrid work is the norm. Healthcare executives can remotely access dashboards and reports of operational performance, utilisation of resources, and budgets during times of war, natural disasters, and pandemics. Having this capability allows hospitals to continue functioning during emergencies or in situations where physical presence is not practical [79].

Cloud-based systems also enable collaboration among healthcare professionals, allowing immediate patient data and medical image sharing. This speeds up the decision-making process and increases the efficiency of diagnosis and treatment. Cloud-based solutions also offer easy integration into other technologies like AI, IoT, and electronic health records (EHR), allowing advanced functionality for telehealth use cases. Cloud computing assists in the uninterrupted and efficient delivery of healthcare services and the elimination of geographical obstacles by allowing for secure, reliable, and accessible on-demand access to hospital data in real time [80].

AUTOMATION AND WORKFLOW OPTIMIZATION

Automation and workflow optimisation are fundamental for improving the efficiency and workflow of healthcare management systems. This reduces manual work, like admin work, giving more time and energy to care providers to care for patients. This helps eliminate errors and lower operational costs. Automation is transforming how healthcare organisations better manage patient data, administrative tasks, and internal workflows with the advancement of technology. Streamlining tasks, including patient intake, discharge, and interdisciplinary interactions, enables improved workflow efficiency and patient satisfaction [81]. Automation and workflow optimisation in HMS are depicted in Fig. (3).

Automation in Administrative Tasks

Most healthcare professionals are forced to endure endless administrative tasks. Implementing automation dramatically improves productivity. Scheduling appointments and managing billing are lengthy processes in the traditional method. Automated systems would take care of these repetitive tasks in an efficient manner, leading to the reduction of errors and a faster turnaround time. Computerised systems can confirm patient data, book appointments, send alerts, and even manage insurance claims, enabling staff to attend to higher-level tasks. Similarly, automation is key to bringing down the costs of labour and boosting the patient experience by reducing waiting times and efficiently managing patient data [82].

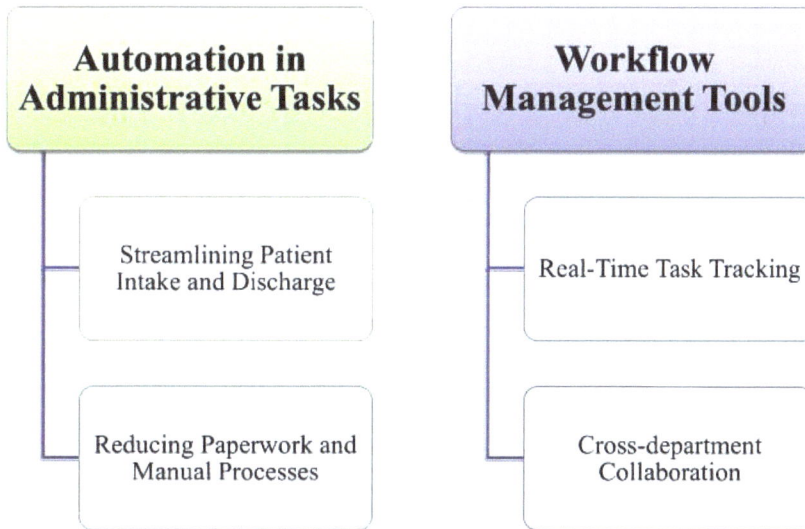

Automation in Administrative Tasks

- Streamlining Patient Intake and Discharge
- Reducing Paperwork and Manual Processes

Workflow Management Tools

- Real-Time Task Tracking
- Cross-department Collaboration

Fig. (3). Automation and workflow optimization in HMS.

Automation in Patient Intake and Discharge

Healthcare providers can reap significant benefits by automating the patient intake and discharge processes. Traditionally, these processes include time-consuming forms and repetitive paperwork, which can open the door to human error, slow turnaround times, and patient dissatisfaction. Using automated systems, patients will be able to fill out forms electronically, taking some of the administrative work off physicians and ensuring proper data collection. Automation can aid in the validation of patient data during intake, similarly to how it can ensure that the data matches what is already on file with the healthcare provider [83].

Before discharge, automation allows for precise follow-up instructions, prescriptions, and appointment reminders to be shared, minimising post-care complications. Such efficiencies are essential but also vastly improve the patient experience by making the flow between inputs seamless. In addition, healthcare providers have real-time access to patient data, leading to better decision-making and more efficient resource allocation. Automating the intake and discharge reduces wait times and facilitates communication, which not only bolsters operational efficiency but also raises patient satisfaction levels significantly [84].

Reducing Paperwork and Manual Processes

The healthcare sector has a lot of redundancies and paper-based workloads, from patient intake forms to medical records, which leads to administrative inefficiencies and errors. Automation solves this problem by digitising the paper trail and reducing manual processes. The use of electronic health records (EHRs) and automated patient registration systems minimizes reliance on paper-based forms, allowing for ease in patient data storage and retrieval solution capabilities. These systems reduce the potential for errors by removing manual data entry methods such as physical record keeping, providing better data stability [85].

It enables quicker insurance claim processing, appointment scheduling, and billing while minimising administrative overheads. In addition, it reduces paper usage, which addresses physical storage and document loss due to damage or misfiling. This helps avoid any unnecessary paperwork and subsequently helps lessen the burden on the environment, too. Automation is making it possible for healthcare providers to divert more of their resources towards patient care and spend less time on administrative work and more on improving healthcare delivery [86].

Workflow Management Tools

Healthcare technology system workflow tools are also vital to operate effectively. Such tools allow healthcare organisations to automate repetitive tasks, manage workflows, and measure progress in real time. By automating administrative responsibilities, patient engagement, departmental communication, and other areas in healthcare facilities can perform seamlessly and save time. Workflow management systems route tasks to the right people, ensure completion in a timely manner, and reduce errors and delays. They also allow for real-time data analysis and enable healthcare providers to conduct informed healthcare decisions regarding resource allocation and patient care, ultimately enhancing performance and patient satisfaction [87].

Real-time Task Tracking

Tracking the movement of tasks in real-time is the key to enhancing the efficiency of healthcare operations. Task-tracking systems are also liberally used to measure the progress of activities occurring in real-time in healthcare facilities. This methodology permits administrators and healthcare workers to seamlessly spot bottlenecks, manage priorities, and deploy resources more efficiently. For instance, in a hospital setting, real-time tracking can monitor the status of medical procedures, patient treatments, or even staff availability [88].

If a task is delayed or not completed as scheduled, real-time alerts can notify supervisors, allowing for swift intervention and adjustments. Task tracking systems also provide transparency by offering data insights into how long tasks take, who is responsible for them, and whether they meet quality standards. This enhances accountability and encourages sustained evolution. Real-time tracking can also streamline inter-departmental communications to ensure seamless patient care delivery by multiple teams. With streamlined task management, they can improve operational efficiency in a way that leads to fewer delays and ultimately improves patient care [89].

Cross-department Collaboration

In a healthcare environment where so many teams must collaborate to deliver comprehensive care, cross-department collaboration is a critical requirement. Communication and efficiency can be improved through workflow optimisation tools that manage department collaboration. For example, when departments such as radiology, surgery, and nursing collaborate seamlessly, the patient journey becomes more integrated, reducing unnecessary delays and improving outcomes. Automation platforms that provide shared access to patient data, treatment plans, and progress updates allow staff members to communicate in real time, ensuring that all teams are aligned and aware of any changes in the patient's condition.

Cross-department collaboration tools help bridge the gap between specialties, leading to enhanced coordination, speed in decision-making, and patient satisfaction. These tools contribute to developing a more patient-centred care environment along with improved efficiency through coordination by breaking down the silos. Additionally, they may minimise miscommunication among departments and engage all relevant departments at each point in the patient care pathway for more accurate diagnoses, timely treatment, and seamless transitions between services of the health system [90, 91].

INTEROPERABILITY OPTIMIZATION

Optimal performance usually requires integration across departments as well as seamless interfacing with external systems. System integration bridges together the different departments of a hospital. Interoperability with outside health systems allows accurate and efficient transfer of information about the patient [92].

System Integration

Hospital system integration refers to integrating separate functions like emergency departments, labs, and other departments that use different systems and bringing them under a single roof. This integration allows for patient data to flow throughout the institution without duplication or error.

Integrating Various Hospital Departments

Incorporating various hospital departments, such as the emergency room (ER), laboratories, and pharmacy, is essential in delivering prompt, coordinated care. Emergency Room departments are established for acute cases, those that require timely treatment, and a mostly integrated interaction between physicians, nurses, and specialists. Through the integration of the ER system with laboratory and pharmacy systems, medical professionals are able to get instant test results, patient histories, and medication orders which speed up diagnosis and treatment plans. Test orders from ER physicians are automatically fed into a laboratory integration system, which minimises delays in generating results. Likewise, pharmacy integration also tracks and delivers prescribed medications without any error, ensuring patient safety. Moreover, system integration facilitates quicker internal communication between the medical staff so that better decisions can be made in less time and contributes towards better resource allocation during such high-pressure situations as trauma care. Integration of care leads to optimisations and reduction of bottlenecks, which, as a result, leads to a better patient experience [93].

Interoperability with External Health Systems

In order to streamline the quality and efficiency of patient care, interoperability with external health systems (*i.e.*, insurance companies and other hospitals) is a key factor. This enables smooth flow of data, ensuring continuity of care between the hospitals and external systems through secure and correct exchange of patient data. Interoperability helps in case the patient is moved from one hospital to another. The hospital that receives the patient will be able to access the medical history, medications, and treatments already undergone and then treat the patient accordingly. Likewise, in communicating with insurance providers, hospitals can easily exchange information on billing and patient data, which enables swift processing of claims and less paperwork cost. Interoperability also improves emergency care situations by allowing rapid access to health records, regardless of location or system. Standardised data formats and protocols, such as HL7 and FHIR, ensure that these systems can understand and process shared data correctly. Interoperability streamlines delays and helps improve patient outcomes, allowing hospitals to communicate with one another as well as other stakeholders like insurers and overall aligning care [94].

Data Exchange Standards

Data exchange standards are necessary for the smooth transfer of health information between information systems and institutions. These standards allow various hospital management systems to communicate efficiently with one another, making sure that data sharing is done appropriately and securely.

Standards for Data Exchange

HL7 (Health Level 7) and FHIR (Fast Healthcare Interoperability Resources) are primary standards required for the unimpeded cross-platform communication of healthcare data in a secure, reliable, and standardised format. HL7 is a framework for the exchange of clinical and administrative data across healthcare settings such as hospitals, insurance companies, and laboratories. That describes a messaging protocol that enables systems to send patient data continuously in a standardised format. As a result, all the technologies have to be able to communicate. HL7 provides several versions, among which fragments of HL7 V2, V3, and, more recently, CDA (Clinical Document Architecture) are commonly used for health information exchange [95].

FHIR is a newer standard developed by HL7 that aims to overcome some of the limitations of previous standards by providing a more flexible and internet-friendly approach to data exchange. FHIR adopts an API approach, allowing systems to query for patient data and return results in an interoperable, real-time format such as JSON and XML. Its modular architecture enables seamless integration with existing solutions, which makes it ideal for mobile health applications, patient portals and external system interoperability. HL7 and FHIR standards ensure that health data remains accurate and able to be accessed across different platforms, minimising errors, improving patient care, and ultimately resulting in a more efficient healthcare delivery system [96].

SECURITY AND PRIVACY IN OPTIMIZING HOSPITAL MANAGEMENT SYSTEMS

One big challenge that needs to be overcome before hospital management systems can reach the status of optimisation is that they need solid security and privacy measures against their patient data. Security includes those mechanisms for protecting data, cybersecurity practices, and healthcare compliance. The security of patient information is crucial. Otherwise, trust will deteriorate, and hackers will pose a threat to patient records. Digital media, as mentioned above, raise privacy issues, so it is essential to continue working on implementing proper access controls and encryption technologies whilst complying with privacy laws and regulations.

Data Security

Data security is the power of protecting patient information in a hospital management system. Personal medical data, such as personal identity, treatment histories, and what has been prescribed to a particular patient, requires special protection from unlawful access and cyber threats. Encryption, as well as secure data storage solutions and access controls, keep patient data safe and private. Encryption alters data into formats that cannot be read in human-readable forms, which ensures that the information remains secure even after a data breach. It is essential to carry out regular audits and updates to the security protocols in place for the system to handle newly emerging threats. Hospitals should adopt a defence-in-depth strategy, combining multiple layers of security, including firewalls, intrusion detection systems, and secure communication channels, to protect data both in transit and at rest [97].

Protecting Sensitive Patient Data Using Encryption

The protection of sensitive patient data also relies heavily on encryption. Encryption turns data that crosses hospital networks, such as patient records, medical history, and billing information, into an unreadable string of text, which can only be decrypted with the appropriate decryption key. By employing encryption on both the transmission and storage levels, hospitals can reduce their risk of data breaches. Encryption secures patient privacy when data transfer is taking place from one department to another, one healthcare provider to another, or one healthcare institution to another. Strong encryption practices also support the protection of data required by privacy laws, such as HIPAA and GDPR, that protect patient data. Cyber threats change over time, so manufacturers should periodically update to protect against new vulnerabilities [98].

Implementing Cybersecurity Measures to Prevent Breaches

Proper cybersecurity is essential to preventing breaches and attacks that target hospital management systems. Healthcare organisations need to implement robust cybersecurity measures that include multi-factor authentication, secure access controls, and regular security updates. Using firewalls, intrusion detection systems (IDS), and intrusion prevention systems (IPS) to detect and block malicious activities. Additionally, staff and clinician education on how to keep the data safe, such as avoiding phishing scams and making sure passwords are strong, is just as critical. Moreover, educating staff and clinicians on best practices for data security, such as avoiding phishing scams and ensuring password strength, is equally important. Hospitals should also regularly back up critical data to ensure business continuity in the event of an attack. Furthermore, they should work with cybersecurity experts to assess for any vulnerabilities or issues and rectify the problems to help reduce the likelihood of data breaches [99].

Compliance with Healthcare Regulations

Compliance with healthcare regulations is essential to maintain the privacy and security of patient data. Compliance is critical because it saves the facilities from paying fines and boosts patients' trust by demonstrating the willingness to protect patients' sensitive data.

HIPAA, GDPR and Other Data Protection Laws

HIPAA and GDPR are among the most recognised regulations in the healthcare space. The Health Insurance Portability and Accountability Act, or HIPAA, requires that healthcare organisations safeguard patient information using physical, administrative, and technical safeguards. It also mandates that healthcare providers keep their data transported over a secured medium and provides patients with control over their health records [100].

Under GDPR, there are stringent data privacy regulations, such as needing to get consent before collecting personal data, maintaining accurate data, and being able to give patients their right to access as well as erase their information. Healthcare organisations are required to adapt their data management practices to comply with these regulations to prevent harsh punishment and protect the confidentiality and integrity of patient data. It obligates these third-party vendors to follow the same privacy laws [101].

Ensuring Secure Data Sharing Across Platforms

One of the significant challenges of hospital management systems is secure data sharing across platforms, as the patient data has to be shared not only between hospitals but also with other healthcare providers and third-party healthcare service providers. To ensure sensitive data is never compromised, hospitals need data exchange protocols like HL7, FHIR, and secure APIs. Eliminating the danger of unauthorised access by ensuring that shared data is encrypted, both in transit and at rest, and that only authorised personnel have access to the data minimises the risk of unauthorised access. Hospitals must ensure their third-party data-sharing agreements comply with healthcare laws, and access and exchanges of data must leave audit trails. Such a secure transfer of data allows seamless patient care without security violations [102].

FUTURE TRENDS IN OPTIMIZING HOSPITAL MANAGEMENT SYSTEMS

The intricate nature of the healthcare facility management process is evolving, with advanced technologies now becoming amalgamated with a hospital management system (HMS). Such systems help automate the workflow, simplify operations, and provide better services to patients. Traditional AI and machine learning automate mundane tasks, enhance the diagnostic process, and assist in forecasting patient outcomes, among other significant trends, flexibility, allowing hospitals to scale up the storage and processing of big data. Blockchain adds security and transparency to data. Mobile apps are quickly becoming an essential tool for improving patient engagement and facilitating patient-provider communication. Such innovations are likely to influence the future of hospital health system management [103].

Robotics in hospital management systems brings greater precision and efficiency while carrying out operational tasks and ensuring safety and accuracy. Robots are now being implemented for some operations, such as stock management, cleaning, and transporting patients. Using automated guided vehicles, hospitals can transport supplies, medications, and even specimens between different departments without expending human effort and making human errors. Suitably robotised cleaning systems will maintain disinfection of frequently touched surfaces and limit the human touch with an infectious agent. In addition to this, sophisticated robotic equipment is hired within an operating room, performing high-precision jobs and leading to shorter rehabilitation periods [104].

5G networks and edge computing are shaping the next-generation hospital management systems. Crucially, 5G also has ultra-low latency and high-speed connectivity, which is a fantastic benefit for the real-time transmission capabilities needed by critical healthcare data. This allows medical devices, patients, and healthcare providers to communicate faster, leading to more efficient decision-making for patient care. In contrast, edge computing processes data close to the data source, where it reduces or builds on the dependency on centralised cloud systems. This acceleration in data processing and real-time analytics comes in handy, especially in cases of emergency care, where time can literally be a matter of life and death. This allows for everything from more intelligent patient monitoring systems to seamless telemedicine and remote diagnostics to be implemented in hospitals utilising 5G and edge computing [105].

CONCLUSION

Optimising the working of Hospital Management Systems (HMS) plays a significant role in enhancing the quality of healthcare, efficiency, and patient outcomes. As healthcare environments become increasingly complex, the traditional approaches to managing them are proving inadequate. HMS optimisation overcomes these challenges by leveraging emerging technology and automating the process *via* better data management. Individual segments associated with patient data management, inventory management, staff management, financial management, *etc.*, can all be hugely potentialised through Artificial Intelligence (AI), Blockchain, Internet of Things (IoT), as well as Cloud Computing. AI is essential for predictive analytics, demand forecasting of resources, and intelligent scheduling, all of which are vital aspects of decision-making. This ensures the security, transparency, and traceability of data, whether in patient records or financial transactions. With asset monitoring and management functionalities, the IoT ecosystem optimises patient care and operational performance. Cloud Computing supports telemedicine through its scalability and remote access features, thus enhancing the general access of hospital facilities. The various departments and other health systems may be easily integrated and interoperable with an HMS, which will help decrease the workload of both medical staff and administrators while improving the patient experience. For smooth integration between the systems, data exchange standards such as HL7 and FHIR are crucial. Looking ahead, future advancements such as robotics for operational tasks and the integration of 5G and edge computing will further revolutionise HMS, making hospitals more agile, responsive, and patient-centred. The optimisation of hospital management systems has become a strategic imperative for healthcare institutions, focusing on better care decision integrity, healthcare efficiency, and overall patient satisfaction.

CONSENT FOR PUBLICATON

All authors have given their consent for publication. The authors authorised Akhil Sharma to handle all correspondence.

ACKNOWLEDGEMENTS

Authors are highly thankful to their Universities/Colleges for providing library facilities for the literature survey.

REFERENCES

[1]   Adebisi OA, Oladosu DA, Busari OA, Oyewola YV. Design and implementation of the hospital management system. Intl J Eng Innov Tech 2015; 5(1): 31-4.

[2]   Ştefan AM, Rusu NR, Ovreiu E, Ciuc M. Empowering healthcare: a comprehensive guide to implementing a robust medical information system—components, benefits, objectives, evaluation criteria, and seamless deployment strategies. App Sys Innov 2024; 7(3): 51.
[http://dx.doi.org/10.3390/asi7030051]

[3]   Kelvin-Agwu MC, Adelodun MO, Igwama GT, Anyanwu EC. Strategies for optimising the management of medical equipment in large healthcare institutions. Strategies 2024; 20(9): 162-70.

[4]   Wadhwa S, Madaan J, Saxena A. Need for flexibility and innovation in healthcare management systems. Global J Flex Syst Manag 2007; 8(1-2): 45-54.
[http://dx.doi.org/10.1007/BF03396519]

[5]   Nishanthan K, Mathyvathana S, Priyanthi R, Thusara A, De Silva DI, Cooray D. The hospital management system. Int J Eng Manag Res 2022; 12(5): 135-49.
[http://dx.doi.org/10.31033/ijemr.12.5.17]

[6]   Javaid M, Haleem A, Singh RP, Suman R. Towards insighting cybersecurity for healthcare domains: A comprehensive review of recent practices and trends. Cyber Security and Applications 2023; 1: 100016.
[http://dx.doi.org/10.1016/j.csa.2023.100016]

[7]   Sharma DP, Lashkari AH, Parizadeh M. Understanding cybersecurity management in healthcare: challenges, strategies and trends. Cham: Springer 2024.

[8]   Ahmad SF, Alam MM, Rahmat MK, *et al.* Leading edge or bleeding edge: Designing a framework for the adoption of a technology in an educational organisation. Sustainability (Basel) 2023; 15(8): 6540.
[http://dx.doi.org/10.3390/su15086540]

[9]   Kumar R, Ansari MT, Baz A, Alhakami H, Agrawal A, Khan RA. A multi-perspective benchmarking framework for estimating usable security of hospital management system software based on fuzzy logic, ANP and TOPSIS methods. Trans Internet Inf Syst (Seoul) 2021; 15(1): 240-63.

[10]   Sarker M. Revolutionizing healthcare: the role of machine learning in the health sector. J Art Intell Gen Sci (JAIGS) 2024; 2(1): 36-61.

[11]   Batun S, Begen MA. Optimisation in healthcare delivery modelling: Methods and applications. In Handbook of Healthcare Operations Management: Methods and Applications 2013 Jan 10 (pp. 75-119). New York, NY: Springer, New York.

[12]   Rechel B, Doyle Y, Grundy E, McKee M. How can health systems respond to population ageing? Copenhagen: World Health Organization 2009.

[13]   Yinusa A, Faezipour M. Optimizing healthcare delivery: a model for staffing, patient assignment, and resource allocation. Applied System Innovation 2023; 6(5): 78.
[http://dx.doi.org/10.3390/asi6050078]

[14]   Adeoye S, Adams R. Leveraging Artificial intelligence for predictive healthcare: a data-driven approach to early diagnosis and personalized treatment. Cogn J Multidis Studies 2024; 4(11): 80-97.
[http://dx.doi.org/10.47760/cognizance.2024.v04i11.006]

[15]   George AS, George AH. Telemedicine: A New Way to Provide Healthcare. Partners Universal Intl Inno J 2023; 1(3): 98-129.

[16]   Junaid SB, Imam AA, Balogun AO, *et al.* Recent advancements in emerging technologies for healthcare management systems: a survey. Healthcare (Basel) 2022; 10(10): 1940.

[17]   Leaven L, Ahmmad K, Peebles D. Inventory management applications for healthcare supply chains. Intel J Sup Chain Manag 2017; 6(3): 1-7.

[18]   Mohamed SA, Mahmoud MA, Mahdi MN, Mostafa SA. Improving efficiency and effectiveness of robotic process automation in human resource management. Sustainability (Basel) 2022; 14(7): 3920.
[http://dx.doi.org/10.3390/su14073920]

[19]   Grath A. The handbook of international trade and finance: the complete guide to risk management, international payments and currency management, bonds and guarantees, credit insurance and trade finance. London: Kogan Page Publishers 2008.

[20]   Nowrozy R. A Security and privacy compliant data sharing solution for healthcare data ecosystems. PhD dissertation. Melbourne: Victoria University 2024.

[21]   Semantha FH, Azam S, Shanmugam B, Yeo KC, Beeravolu AR. A conceptual framework to ensure

privacy in patient record management system. IEEE Access 2021; 9: 165667-89.
[http://dx.doi.org/10.1109/ACCESS.2021.3134873]

[22] Wu P, Nam MY, Choi J, Kirlik A, Sha L, Berlin RB Jr. Supporting emergency medical care teams with an integrated status display providing real-time access to medical best practices, workflow tracking, and patient data. J Med Syst 2017; 41(12): 186.
[http://dx.doi.org/10.1007/s10916-017-0829-x] [PMID: 29039621]

[23] Reddy A, Ghantasala GP, Kurra M, Ayyappa RM. Patient empowerment through secure data management. In: Using Blockchain Technology in Healthcare Settings. CRC Press 2025 Mar 24; pp. 153-174. [https://doi.org/10.2196/60562]

[24] Băjenaru OL, Băjenaru L, Ianculescu M, Constantin VȘ, Gușatu AM, Nuță CR. Geriatric healthcare supported by decision-making tools integrated into digital health solutions. Electronics (Basel) 2024; 13(17): 3440.
[http://dx.doi.org/10.3390/electronics13173440]

[25] Singh S, Pankaj B, Nagarajan K, Singh NP, Bala V. Blockchain with cloud for handling healthcare data: A privacy-friendly platform. Mater Today Proc 2022; 62: 5021-6.
[http://dx.doi.org/10.1016/j.matpr.2022.04.910]

[26] Fareed M, Yassin AA. Privacy-preserving multi-factor authentication and role-based access control scheme for the E-healthcare system. Bull Elect Eng Inform 2022; 11(4): 2131-41.
[http://dx.doi.org/10.11591/eei.v11i4.3658]

[27] Dinh-Le C, Chuang R, Chokshi S, Mann D. Wearable health technology and electronic health record integration: scoping review and future directions. JMIR Mhealth Uhealth 2019; 7(9): e12861.
[http://dx.doi.org/10.2196/12861] [PMID: 31512582]

[28] Adebanjo D, Laosirihongthong T, Samaranayake P. Prioritizing lean supply chain management initiatives in healthcare service operations: a fuzzy AHP approach. Prod Plann Contr 2016; 27(12): 953-66.
[http://dx.doi.org/10.1080/09537287.2016.1164909]

[29] Ahmad RW, Salah K, Jayaraman R, Yaqoob I, Omar M, Ellahham S. Blockchain-based forward supply chain and waste management for COVID-19 medical equipment and supplies. IEEE Access 2021; 9: 44905-27.
[http://dx.doi.org/10.1109/ACCESS.2021.3066503] [PMID: 34812386]

[30] Ting SL, Kwok SK, Tsang AHC, Lee WB. Critical elements and lessons learnt from the implementation of an RFID-enabled healthcare management system in a medical organization. J Med Syst 2011; 35(4): 657-69.
[http://dx.doi.org/10.1007/s10916-009-9403-5] [PMID: 20703523]

[31] Ahmadi E, Masel DT, Hostetler S, Maihami R, Ghalehkhondabi I. A centralised stochastic inventory control model for perishable products considering age-dependent purchase price and lead time: Span Soc Stat Oper Res. 2020 Apr; 28(1): 231-69.

[32] Hinkka V, Tätilä J. RFID tracking implementation model for the technical trade and construction supply chains. Autom Construct 2013; 35: 405-14.
[http://dx.doi.org/10.1016/j.autcon.2013.05.024]

[33] Aldahiri A, Alrashed B, Hussain W. Trends in using IoT with machine learning in health prediction system. Forecasting 2021; 3(1): 181-206.
[http://dx.doi.org/10.3390/forecast3010012]

[34] Smith AD, Flanegin FR. E-procurement and automatic identification: enhancing supply chain management in the healthcare industry. Int J Electron Healthc 2004; 1(2): 176-98.
[http://dx.doi.org/10.1504/IJEH.2004.005866] [PMID: 18048219]

[35] Nwosu NT. Reducing operational costs in healthcare through advanced BI tools and data integration. World J Adv Res Rev 2024; 22(3): 1144-56.

[http://dx.doi.org/10.30574/wjarr.2024.22.3.1774]

[36]   Rehman A, Naz S, Razzak I. Leveraging big data analytics in healthcare enhancement: trends, challenges and opportunities. Multimedia Syst 2022; 28(4): 1339-71.
[http://dx.doi.org/10.1007/s00530-020-00736-8]

[37]   Azmy A, Hermawan E, Arifin AL, Pranogyo AB. The effect of talent management optimisation on workforce agility through job satisfaction and employee engagement to develop excellent service in private hospitals. Acad Strat Manag J 2022; 21(5): 1-20.

[38]   Do MH, Bui TTH, Phan T, *et al.* Strengthening public health management capacity in Vietnam: preparing local public health workers for new roles in a decentralised health system. J Public Health Manag Pract 2018; 24 (Suppl. 2): S74-81.
[http://dx.doi.org/10.1097/PHH.0000000000000755] [PMID: 29369260]

[39]   Massarweh L. Readiness for improving safe care delivery through web-based hospital nurse scheduling & staffing technology: a multi-hospital approach. Doctor of Nursing Practice project. Spokane (WA): Gonzaga University; 2017.

[40]   Barrera-Cámara RA, Canepa-Sáenz AA. Artificial intelligence and applications in drinking water management. In: Smart Water Technology for Sustainable Management in Modern Cities. IGI Global Scientific Publishing 2025; pp. 285-306.
[http://dx.doi.org/10.4018/979-8-3693-8074-1.ch012]

[41]   Menon S, George A, Mathew N, Vivek V, John J. Smart workplace—Using iBeacon. In: International Conference on Networks & Advances in Computational Technologies (NetACT) 2017; 396-400.

[42]   Erickson SM, Rockwern B, Koltov M, McLean RM. Medical Practice and Quality Committee of the American College of Physicians*. Putting patients first by reducing administrative tasks in health care: a position paper of the American College of Physicians. Ann Intern Med 2017; 166(9): 659-61.
[http://dx.doi.org/10.7326/M16-2697] [PMID: 28346948]

[43]   Pieneman-Elbers DC. Building a learning healthcare system: a path to optimising big health data to inform clinical care decisions. PhD dissertation. Burlington (VT): The University of Vermont and State Agricultural College 2022.

[44]   Varma A, Budhwar PS, DeNisi A. Performance management around the globe: introduction and agenda. In: Varma A, Budhwar PS, DeNisi A, Eds. Performance management systems. 1st ed. London: Routledge; 2008. pp. 15-39.
[http://dx.doi.org/10.4324/9780203885673-2]

[45]   Atkins G, Davies N, Wilkinson F, Guerin B, Pope T, Tetlow G. Performance Tracker 2019. Institute for Government 2019; (Nov): 118.

[46]   Chow-Chua C, Goh M. Framework for evaluating performance and quality improvement in hospitals. Manag Serv Qual 2002; 12(1): 54-66.
[http://dx.doi.org/10.1108/09604520210415399]

[47]   Atluri H, Thummisetti BS. Optimising revenue cycle management in healthcare: a comprehensive analysis of the charge navigator system. Intel Num J Mach Learn Robots 2023; 7(7): 1-3.

[48]   Ranjan P, Soman S, Ateria AK, Srivastava PK. Streamlining payment workflows using a patient wallet for hospital information systems. In: 2018 IEEE 31st International Symposium on Computer-Based Medical Systems (CBMS).Karlstad, Sweden. IEEE; 2018. pp. 339–44.
[http://dx.doi.org/10.1109/CBMS.2018.00066]

[49]   Bhuvana R, Hemalatha RJ, Baskar S, Kosalaram K. Introduction to smart hospital. In: Tyagi AK, Ed. Artificial intelligence-enabled blockchain technology and digital twin for smart hospitals. Hoboken (NJ): Wiley 2024. pp. 1–24.
[http://dx.doi.org/10.1002/9781394287420.ch1]

[50]   Murala DK, Panda SK, Dash SP. MedMetaverse: the medical care of chronic disease patients and managing data using artificial intelligence, blockchain, and wearable devices state-of-the-art

methodology. IEEE Access 2023; 11: 138954-85.
[http://dx.doi.org/10.1109/ACCESS.2023.3340791]

[51] Machireddy JR. Revolutionizing claims processing in the healthcare industry: the expanding role of automation and AI. Hong Kong J of AI and Med 2022; 2(1): 10-36.

[52] Manirabona A, Fourati LC, Boudjit S. Investigation on healthcare monitoring systems: Innovative services and applications In: Wearable technologies: Concepts, methodologies, tools, and applications. IGI Global 2018; pp. 1264-83.

[53] Mandal S, Kumar M, Bhumika K, Ali S, Jahan I, Mandal S. Impact of electronic health records and automation on pharmaceutical management efficiency: a narrative review. Intel J Heal Sci Eng. 2025 Feb 17:21-36.

[54] Al Tahaivan MS, Al Buzobdah AH, Al Yami MY, *et al.* Evaluating efficacy: a critical review of innovative strategies In: optimizing patient care within health services and hospital management. J Surv Fish Sci 2023; 10(5): 69-74.

[55] Olaoye F, Potter K. Optimizing healthcare operations with AI-driven decision support systems. EasyChair Preprint 12832. EasyChair 2024.

[56] Prabhod KJ. The role of artificial intelligence in reducing healthcare costs and improving operational efficiency. Quart J Eme Techno Innov 2024; 9(2): 47-59.

[57] Ali H. AI for pandemic preparedness and infectious disease surveillance: predicting outbreaks, modelling transmission, and optimising public health interventions. Int J Res Publ Rev 2024; 5(8): 4605-19.

[58] Niyonambaza I, Zennaro M, Uwitonze A. Predictive maintenance (Pdm) structure using Internet of things (IoT) for mechanical equipment used in hospitals in Rwanda. Future Internet 2020; 12(12): 224.
[http://dx.doi.org/10.3390/fi12120224]

[59] Amiri Z. Leveraging AI-enabled information systems for healthcare management. J Comp Info Sys. 2024 Oct 17: 1-28.

[60] Aman Z, Qidwai MA. Role of artificial intelligence in strengthening healthcare systems. In: Qidwai MA, Ed. Intersection of human rights and AI in healthcare. Hershey, PA: IGI Global Scientific Publishing 2025; pp. 253–82.

[61] Singh B, Gupta A. Blockchain technology for hospital management: a visualisation and review of research trends. In: 2021 2nd International Conference on Smart Electronics and Communication (ICOSEC). Trichy, India. New York: IEEE 2021; pp. 395–9.
[http://dx.doi.org/10.1109/ICOSEC51865.2021.9591880]

[62] Zaabar B, Cheikhrouhou O, Jamil F, Ammi M, Abid M. HealthBlock: A secure blockchain-based healthcare data management system. Comput Netw 2021; 200: 108500.
[http://dx.doi.org/10.1016/j.comnet.2021.108500]

[63] Yue X, Wang H, Jin D, Li M, Jiang W. Healthcare data gateways: found healthcare intelligence on blockchain with novel privacy risk control. J Med Syst 2016; 40(10): 218.
[http://dx.doi.org/10.1007/s10916-016-0574-6] [PMID: 27565509]

[64] Yaqoob I, Salah K, Jayaraman R, Al-Hammadi Y. Blockchain for healthcare data management: opportunities, challenges, and future recommendations. Neural Comput Appl 2022; 34(14): 11475-90.
[http://dx.doi.org/10.1007/s00521-020-05519-w]

[65] Abrahams TO, Farayola OA, Kaggwa S, Uwaoma PU, Hassan AO, Dawodu SO. Reviewing third-party risk management: best practices in accounting and cybersecurity for superannuation organizations. Finan Account Res J 2024; 6(1): 21-39.
[http://dx.doi.org/10.51594/farj.v6i1.706]

[66] Said HE, Al Barghuthi NB, Badi SM, Girija S. Design of a blockchain-based patient record tracking system. International Conference on IoT and Health Cham: Springer Nature Switzerland 2023; pp.

145-161.

[67]   Velmovitsky PE, Bublitz FM, Fadrique LX, Morita PP. Blockchain applications in health care and public health: increased transparency. JMIR Med Inform 2021; 9(6): e20713.
[http://dx.doi.org/10.2196/20713] [PMID: 34100768]

[68]   Thangaraj M, Ponmalar PP, Anuradha S. Internet of Things (IoT) enabled innovative autonomous hospital management system: real-world healthcare use case with the technology drivers. In: 2015 IEEE International Conference on Computational Intelligence and Computing Research (ICCIC). Coimbatore, India: IEEE 2015; pp. 1–8.

[69]   Gourisaria MK, Agrawal R, Singh V, Rautaray SS, Pandey M. AI and IoT enabled innovative hospital management systems. In Data Science in Societal Applications: Concepts and Implications Singapore: Springer Nature 2022; pp. 77-106.

[70]   Mamdiwar SD, R A, Shakruwala Z, Chadha U, Srinivasan K, Chang CY. Recent advances in IoT-assisted wearable sensor systems for healthcare monitoring. Biosensors (Basel) 2021; 11(10): 372.
[http://dx.doi.org/10.3390/bios11100372] [PMID: 34677328]

[71]   Michalska K. IoT-enabled smart pharmacy automation systems for medication dispensing. African. J Artif Intell Sust Devel 2024; 4(2): 36-43.

[72]   Raikar AS, Kumar P, Raikar GVS, Somnache SN. Advances and challenges in IoT-based smart drug delivery systems: a comprehensive review. Applied System Innovation 2023; 6(4): 62.
[http://dx.doi.org/10.3390/asi6040062]

[73]   Pradhan B, Bhattacharyya S, Pal K. IoT-based applications in healthcare devices. J Healthc Eng 2021; 2021(1): 6632599.
[PMID: 33791084]

[74]   Kong HJ, An S, Lee S, *et al.* Usage of the internet of things in medical institutions and its implications. Healthc Inform Res 2022; 28(4): 287-96.
[http://dx.doi.org/10.4258/hir.2022.28.4.287] [PMID: 36380426]

[75]   Shanmugasundaram G, Thiyagarajan P, Janaki A. A survey of Cloud-based healthcare monitoring systems for hospital management. In Proceedings of the International Conference on Data Engineering and Communication Technology: ICDECT. Singapore: Springer 2017; pp. 549-557.

[76]   Aceto G, Persico V, Pescapé A. Industry 4.0 and health: Internet of things, big data, and cloud computing for healthcare 4.0. J Ind Inf Integr 2020; 18: 100129.
[http://dx.doi.org/10.1016/j.jii.2020.100129]

[77]   Boda VV, Allam H. Ready for anything: disaster recovery strategies every healthcare IT team should know. Int J Emerg Trends Comput Sci Inf Technol 2022; 3(1): 38–46.

[78]   Ahmed S, Raja MY. Virtual hospitals: integration of telemedicine, healthcare services, and cloud computing. In: Eren H, Webster JG, Eds. Telemedicine and Electronic Medicine. Boca Raton (FL): CRC Press 2018; p. 51–72.

[79]   Dang LM, Piran MJ, Han D, Min K, Moon H. A survey on the Internet of Things and cloud computing for healthcare. Electronics (Basel) 2019; 8(7): 768.
[http://dx.doi.org/10.3390/electronics8070768]

[80]   Kanagaraj G, Sumathi AC. Proposal of an open-source cloud computing system for exchanging medical images of a hospital information system. In 3rd International Conference on Trendz in Information Sciences & Computing (TISC2011) 2011 Dec 8 (pp. 144-149). IEEE.
[http://dx.doi.org/10.1109/TISC.2011.6169102]

[81]   Zayas-Cabán T, Haque SN, Kemper N. Identifying opportunities for workflow automation in health care: lessons learned from other industries. Appl Clin Inform 2021; 12(3): 686-97.
[http://dx.doi.org/10.1055/s-0041-1731744] [PMID: 34320683]

[82]   Nayak A, Satpathy I, Patnaik BC, Gujrati R, Uygun H. Simplified hospital management system:

Robotic Process Automation (RPA) to rescue In: Data-centric AI solutions and emerging technologies in the healthcare ecosystem. CRC Press 2024; pp. 281-302.

[83]   Falcetta FS, de Almeida FK, Lemos JCS, Goldim JR, da Costa CA. Automatic documentation of professional health interactions: A systematic review. Artif Intell Med 2023; 137: 102487.
[http://dx.doi.org/10.1016/j.artmed.2023.102487] [PMID: 36868684]

[84]   Oloruntoba Babawarun , Rawlings Chidi , Chidi R, Adeniyi AO, Okolo CA. A comprehensive review of data analytics in healthcare management: Leveraging big data for decision-making. World J Adv Res Rev 2024; 21(2): 1810-21.
[http://dx.doi.org/10.30574/wjarr.2024.21.2.0590]

[85]   Pillai AS. AI-enabled hospital management systems for modern healthcare: an analysis of system components and interdependencies J Adv Anal Health Manag 2023; 7(1): 212-28.

[86]   Uchechukwu BN, Ohinameuwa A. Enhanced health (record) information management system using mobile application development framework. J Sci Technol 2025; 30(3): 92-107.

[87]   Zhai K, Yousef MS, Mohammed S, Al-Dewik NI, Qoronfleh MW. Optimising clinical workflow using precision medicine and advanced data analytics. Processes (Basel) 2023; 11(3): 939.
[http://dx.doi.org/10.3390/pr11030939]

[88]   Islam M, Rashid S, Rafid L, Badrul T, Islam A, Chaudhry BM. Design and Evaluation of a Smartwatch-Based Physiological Signal-Driven Workplace Stress Management mHealth Tool for Bangladeshi Healthcare Professionals. In 2024 Advances in Science and Engineering Technology International Conferences (ASET) 2024 Jun 3 (pp. 1-10).
[http://dx.doi.org/10.1109/ASET60340.2024.10708713]

[89]   Adenova G, Kausova G, Saliev T, *et al.* Optimization of radiology diagnostic services for patients with stroke in multidisciplinary hospitals. Mater Sociomed 2024; 36(3): 160-72.
[http://dx.doi.org/10.5455/msm.2024.36.160-172] [PMID: 39712327]

[90]   Liu C, Li H, Zhang S, Cheng L, Zeng Q. Cross-department collaborative healthcare process model discovery from event logs. IEEE Trans Autom Sci Eng 2023; 20(3): 2115-25.
[http://dx.doi.org/10.1109/TASE.2022.3194312]

[91]   Rahman MH, Hossain MD, Uddin MK, Hossan KM. The future of healthcare: Exploring the creative integration of cloud computing For enhanced e-health solutions. SSRN 5041530.2024;
[http://dx.doi.org/10.2139/ssrn.5041530]

[92]   Alrajeh NA, Elmir B, Bounabat B, El Hami N. Interoperability optimization in healthcare collaboration networks. Biomed Tech (Berl) 2012; 57(5): 403-11.
[http://dx.doi.org/10.1515/bmt-2011-0118] [PMID: 25854667]

[93]   Avula R. Overcoming data silos in healthcare with strategies for enhancing integration and interoperability to improve clinical and operational efficiency. Journal of Advanced Analytics in Healthcare Management 2020; 4(10): 26-44.

[94]   MacAdam K. Interoperability and the path to comprehensive health information exchange. NYU Ann Surv Am L 2020; 76: 743.

[95]   Gazzarata R, Almeida J, Lindsköld L, *et al.* HL7 Fast Healthcare Interoperability Resources (HL7 FHIR) in digital healthcare ecosystems for chronic disease management: Scoping review. Int J Med Inform 2024; 189: 105507.
[http://dx.doi.org/10.1016/j.ijmedinf.2024.105507] [PMID: 38870885]

[96]   Bender D, Sartipi K. HL7 FHIR: an agile and RESTful approach to healthcare information exchange. In: Proceedings of the 26th IEEE International Symposium on Computer-Based Medical Systems. Porto, Portugal. New York: IEEE 2013; pp. 326–31.
[http://dx.doi.org/10.1109/CBMS.2013.6627810]

[97]   Isibor E. Regulation of healthcare data security: Legal obligations in a digital age. SSRN 4957244.2024;

[http://dx.doi.org/10.2139/ssrn.4957244]

[98]   Goyal P, Sharma P, Sharma M, Pareek A. The importance of data encryption in data security. J Nonlinear Ana Optimiz 2023; 13(1): 01-11.
[http://dx.doi.org/10.36893/JNAO.2022.V13I02.001-011]

[99]   Argaw ST, Troncoso-Pastoriza JR, Lacey D, *et al.* Cybersecurity of Hospitals: discussing the challenges and working towards mitigating the risks. BMC Med Inform Decis Mak 2020; 20(1): 146.
[http://dx.doi.org/10.1186/s12911-020-01161-7] [PMID: 32620167]

[100]   Syed FM. ES FK. Ensuring HIPAA and GDPR Compliance Through Advanced IAM Analytics. Int J Adv Eng Technol Innov 2018; 1(2): 71-94.

[101]   Mondschein CF, Monda C. The EU's General Data Protection Regulation (GDPR) in a research context. In: Kubben P, Dumontier M, Dekker A, Eds. Fundamentals of Clinical Data Science. Cham: Springer 2019; p. 55–71.

[102]   Oliveira NR, Santos YR, Mendes ACR, *et al.* Storage standards and solutions, data storage, sharing, and structuring in digital health: A Brazilian case study. Information (Basel) 2023; 15(1): 20.
[http://dx.doi.org/10.3390/info15010020]

[103]   Arisha A, Rashwan W. Modeling of healthcare systems: past, current and future trends. In: 2016 Winter Simulation Conference (WSC). Washington, DC, USA. New York: IEEE 2016; pp. 1523–34.
[http://dx.doi.org/10.1109/WSC.2016.7822203]

[104]   Hussain SJ, Thangavel S, Kumar A. Enhancing hospital management through robotics. In: Bansal P, Kumar R, Kumar A, Dasig DD Jr, Eds. Artificial intelligence and communication techniques in industry 5.0. Boca Raton (FL): CRC Press 2025; p. 373.
[http://dx.doi.org/10.1201/9781003494027-24]

[105]   Bishoyi PK, Misra S. Enabling green mobile-edge computing for 5G-based healthcare applications. IEEE Trans Green Commun Netw 2021; 5(3): 1623-31.
[http://dx.doi.org/10.1109/TGCN.2021.3075903]

CHAPTER 3

Health Information Exchange (HIE) for Seamless Data Sharing

Shaweta Sharma[1], Akhil Sharma[2], Sunita[2], Akanksha Sharma[2], Ashish Verma[3] and Geetika Goel[4,*]

[1] *School of Medical and Allied Sciences, Galgotias University, Yamuna Expressway, Gautam Buddha Nagar, Uttar Pradesh 201310, India*

[2] *R.J. College of Pharmacy, Raipur, Gharbara, Tappal, Khair, Uttar Pradesh 202165, India*

[3] *Mangalmay Pharmacy College, Greater Noida, Uttar Pradesh 201306, India*

[4] *Motherhood University, village karoundi, bhagwanpur, Roorkee, Uttarakhand 247661, India*

Abstract: Health Information Exchange (HIE) is a novel method to modernise healthcare by synchronising electronic health data sharing among healthcare providers, organisations and stakeholders. This chapter examines the utilisation of HIE as a foundation for more successful patient, quality and value-based healthcare delivery. The chapter begins by defining HIE and outlining its scope, encompassing the seamless integration of disparate healthcare systems, including electronic health records (EHRs) and laboratory and imaging platforms, through interoperability standards such as HL7 and FHIR. It analyses the benefits of HIE, *i.e.*, enhanced care coordination, reduced redundancy with diagnostic test orders, increased patient safety, and patients' access to self-serving medical records in detail. Technological advancements driving HIE, such as blockchain for data security, artificial intelligence for predictive analytics, and cloud computing for scalable storage, are discussed alongside the critical implementation challenges, including data standardisation, privacy concerns, and adoption barriers. The chapter further discusses the role of HIE in addressing healthcare disparities, especially in medically underserved areas, and its impact on public health efforts and research. The chapter provides case studies and uses cases to exhibit the success of HIE in augmenting healthcare delivery while also saving money. Finally, it imagines a future where HIE, driven by new technologies and shared policies, becomes the cornerstone of an interconnected and patient-centric healthcare world. This chapter underscores HIE's pivotal role in revolutionising healthcare by leveraging technology for efficiency and accessibility.

Keywords: Blockchain technology, Data security, Electronic Health Records (EHR), Healthcare efficiency, Health Information Exchange (HIE), Interoperability, Patient empowerment.

---

* **Corresponding author Geetika Goel:** Motherhood University, village karoundi, bhagwanpur, Roorkee, Uttarakhand 247661, India; E-mail: Geetikagoel89@gmail.com

INTRODUCTION

Health Information Exchange (HIE) is the secure, real-time, electronic sharing of patient and population-level information among healthcare providers, organisations, and stakeholders to optimise healthcare delivery quality, safety, and efficiency. By facilitating the seamless flow of health information, HIE allows healthcare professionals to access the most current and exact patient information if or as needed, allowing for smooth health information movement. This facilitates well-informed decisions, minimises medical errors, avoids excessive tests and other wasteful healthcare resources, and optimises patient outcomes. The HIE serves as the infrastructure for interoperability, connecting disparate healthcare silos [1, 2].

Health Information Exchange is a broad, transformative healthcare and data management area. Fundamentally, HIE is about promoting interoperability, which means that data systems such as Electronic Health Records (EHRs), laboratory systems, imaging platforms, and other providers of patient health information can successfully exchange data in standardised formats such as HL7, FHIR or DICOM [3]. The software program helps coordinate care between primary care providers, specialists, pharmacists, and emergency services in critical transition periods to prevent information gaps from compromising patient safety. HIE supports public health by creating epidemic surveillance and outbreak monitoring, and supporting large-scale epidemiological studies by providing aggregated, de-identified data. It empowers patients by granting them access to their health records through patient portals or mobile applications, fostering active participation in their healthcare journey and improving health literacy [4, 5].

Furthermore, HIE plays a critical role in achieving cost-saving in healthcare by preventing duplication of tests, minimising administrative redundancies, and increasing operational efficiency. Promoting equity and accessibility paves the way for healthcare delivery in underprivileged or remote areas *via* telehealth platforms, networked data sharing, and better specialist connectivity. HIEs operate through varied models appropriate for specific organisations and regional needs. A centralised model consolidates data into a central repository, providing a single access point but requiring robust security measures. In a decentralised model, data is kept with source systems, and data sharing on demand is enabled, securing capabilities over the cloud but at the cost of potentially slower application performance. A hybrid model combines the benefits of both, balancing efficiency, scalability, and security [6, 7].

HIE is more than data sharing on a technical level. It addresses regulatory compliance beyond privacy laws such as HIPAA and GDPR, fosters stakeholder collaboration, and takes HIE to the next level by integrating blockchain, AI, and cloud, which would enhance its efficacy. With these abilities, HIE emerges as a key enabler for a connected and efficient patient-centered healthcare ecosystem [8].

IMPORTANCE OF HIE IN MODERN HEALTHCARE

Health Information Exchange (HIE) is crucial to modern-day healthcare. That enables the seamless exchange of patient information among different stakeholders, improving care coordination and ensuring that patients receive high-quality, timely care. HIE reduces medical errors and provides appropriate forms with real-time patient information to healthcare providers, avoiding duplication of test results and enhancing patient safety. It, moreover, diminishes healthcare expenses when it takes away peevishly agreed-upon medical procedures and administrative inefficiency [9, 10].

Furthermore, HIE enables patient control by allowing patients access to their health data from a consumer-facing application, promoting transparency, and taking an active role in their care. This engagement of the patient results in better health outcomes where patients are more educated and invested in their treatment choices. In addition to its importance in emergencies and complex care, HIE is essential for giving clinicians actionable information at the point of clinical need (timely, evidence-based care) and provides aggregated data for effective public health [11].

It fills the gap in healthcare deemed to be beyond some remote locations or underserved areas by providing state-of-the-art technology for consulting remotely with individuals residing that far away. HIE helps meet legal and regulatory requirements for health information privacy while maintaining data security and appropriately sharing patient data. Ultimately, HIE is indispensable for more efficient and cost-effective healthcare systems, leading to better care delivery and patient security and achieving a well-integrated, patient-centred health system [12 - 14].

GOALS OF HIE

The goals of Health Information Exchange (HIE) are centred around improving healthcare delivery, enhancing patient outcomes, and optimising the overall efficiency of healthcare systems. Fig. (1) describes the key goals of health information exchange.

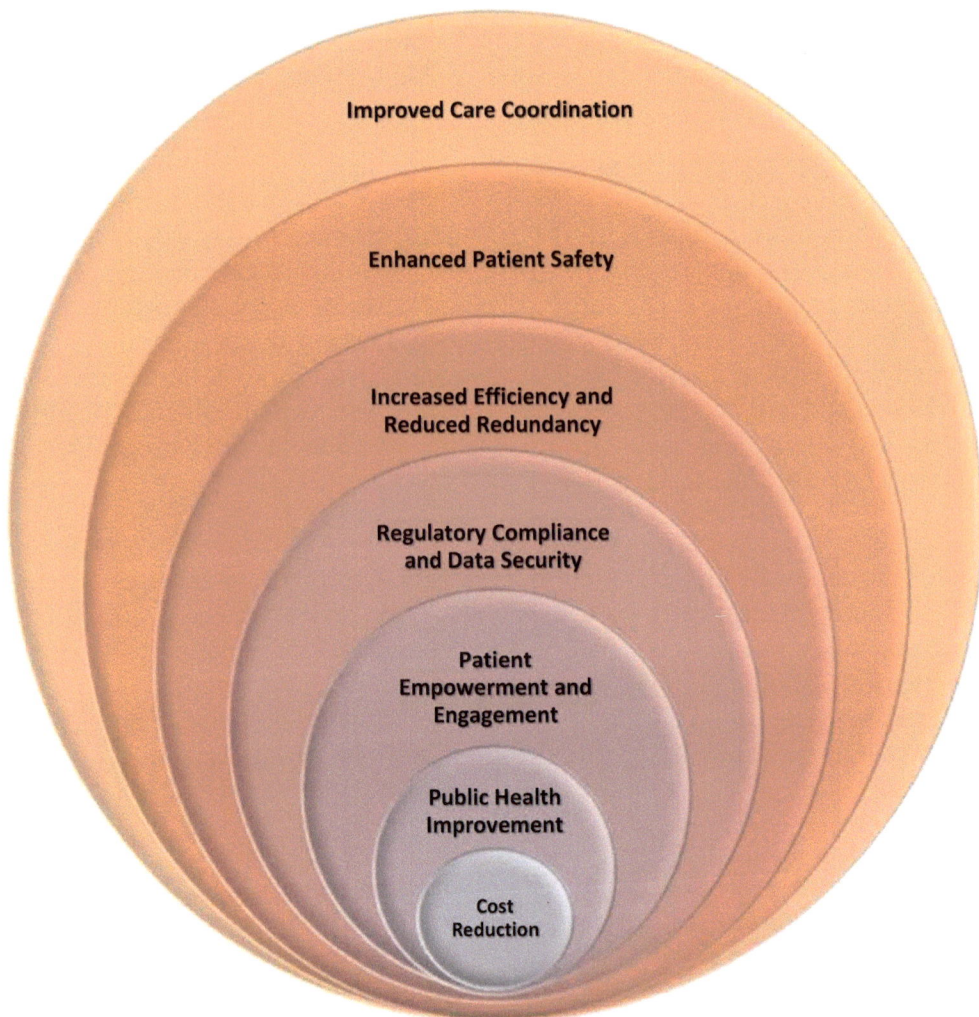

Fig. (1). Goals of health information exchange (HIE).

Improved Care Coordination

The primary purpose of HIE is to improve care coordination among healthcare providers, which means ensuring that patients receive holistic and timely treatment across various healthcare settings. HIE enables healthcare professionals (primary care physicians, emergency care providers, specialists, hospitals, *etc.*) to access a patient's comprehensive medical history, past treatments, lab tests, and prescriptions. This real-time exchange of information ensures care teams have a comprehensive perspective on the patient's health status, mitigating potential gaps in care. HIE allows those specialists to share their thoughts based on similar information and work together towards one strategy of care, so there are fewer breaks or duplications in a patient continuum of care. In particular, care coordination for managing chronic disease, elderly patients, and hospital-to-home can be continuity, and communication is essential to prevent avoidable complications [15 - 17].

Enhanced Patient Safety

HIE dramatically enhances patient safety by reducing the dangers of incomplete or inaccurate information. Ultimately, having fully transparent and real-time health data allows healthcare providers to avoid decisions based on partial or stale information. This minimises medical errors like wrong medicines, drug rounds, or incorrect diagnoses. For example, when a patient rolls up at the emergency department, clinicians can see the patient's allergies, previous trips, and current drugs. This might highlight dangerous interactions between medicines or regular allergies that may have been missed. In addition, HIE helps lower the probability of redundant tests and procedures that can put patients in danger and unnecessarily raise medical costs [18 - 20].

Increased Efficiency and Reduced Redundancy

HIE helps healthcare systems become more efficient by improving workflows, reducing duplicate medical procedures, and coordinating patient care. Some examples include if a patient has already received a specific diagnostic test or imaging study, the HIE allows healthcare providers to access those results without duplicating orders, which lowers time and costs. Using real-time data, healthcare providers can instantly retrieve prior tests, diagnoses, and treatment plans, which improves turnaround time for care delivery and prevents patients from undergoing redundant procedures. It also helps reduce the administrative load of getting patient data from one healthcare provider to another in writing, copying, faxing or in person. This translates into a leaner, meaner, and more cost-effective system of care [21 - 23].

Cost Reduction

HIE also helps lower healthcare costs by improving efficiency and reducing redundancy. Healthcare organisations can save substantial costs by eliminating duplicate tests, procedures, and unnecessary hospital admissions. For example, accessing a patient's medical records, including imaging results and lab reports, through an HIE instead of repeating these tests in various healthcare settings- can save money and time. Moreover, HIE streamlines administrative tasks such as billing, insurance claims, and medical records management, thereby decreasing the operational costs. The benefits of HIE to the healthcare community in terms of overall cost reductions, and the sustainability of healthcare systems by enhancing resource utilisation are making healthcare more accessible [24 - 26].

Patient Empowerment and Engagement

HIE enables patient empowerment by allowing them to access their health records and encouraging them to participate actively in healthcare decisions. When we provide patients with the tools to view their records through online portals or mobile apps, they can see visit notes themselves (if available) and look at medical history and lab results, medications and treatment plans, which can help them have more informed conversations with their healthcare provider. This provision helps patients manage their health better, make more informed decisions and follow through on their prescribed treatment plans. Empowered patients are also more likely to engage in prevention services and health management while having chronic disease and seek care when appropriate, contributing to better clinical outcomes. In addition, HIE contributes to a more collaborative, patient-centred care environment by increasing transparency and trust in the healthcare system [27 - 29].

Public Health Improvement

HIE is a key contributor to advancing public health through data needed for disease surveillance, epidemiological research, and population health monitoring. HIE shares patient information collected from one provider to other health authorities, enabling the tracing of disease patterns and outbreak alerts, and assessing whether they are effective. During health crises like the current COVID-19 pandemic, real-time data sharing over HIEs has proved invaluable for monitoring cases, coordinating responses, and carrying out containment actions. HIE also encourages research by making de-identified patient information available in studies to better understand disease patterns, treatment effectiveness, and healthcare results. In doing so, HIE supports individual patient care and the more significant public health picture in managing and avoiding large-scale health problems [30 - 33].

Regulatory Compliance and Data Security

Ensuring compliance with healthcare regulations is a crucial goal of HIE. Health Information Exchange platforms must conform to high legal standards for securing sensitive health data and patient privacy. Through secure, encrypted data exchange protocols and transparency in patient information use, HIE is responsible for enabling and enforcing healthcare providers to comply with such laws. These steps help to mitigate the chances of data leaks and have saved patients from losing their privacy. HIE provides a legal and secure way of exchanging health data over the Internet; it helps build trust between healthcare providers and patients and facilitates in maintaining a legally compliant atmosphere for sharing information [34, 35].

COMPONENTS OF HIE

HIE comprises several key components, which are summarised in Fig. (**2**), that work together to ensure the efficient, secure, and seamless sharing of patient data across various healthcare systems and organisations. These components are essential for enabling interoperability, improving care coordination, and enhancing healthcare delivery. The main components of HIE include:

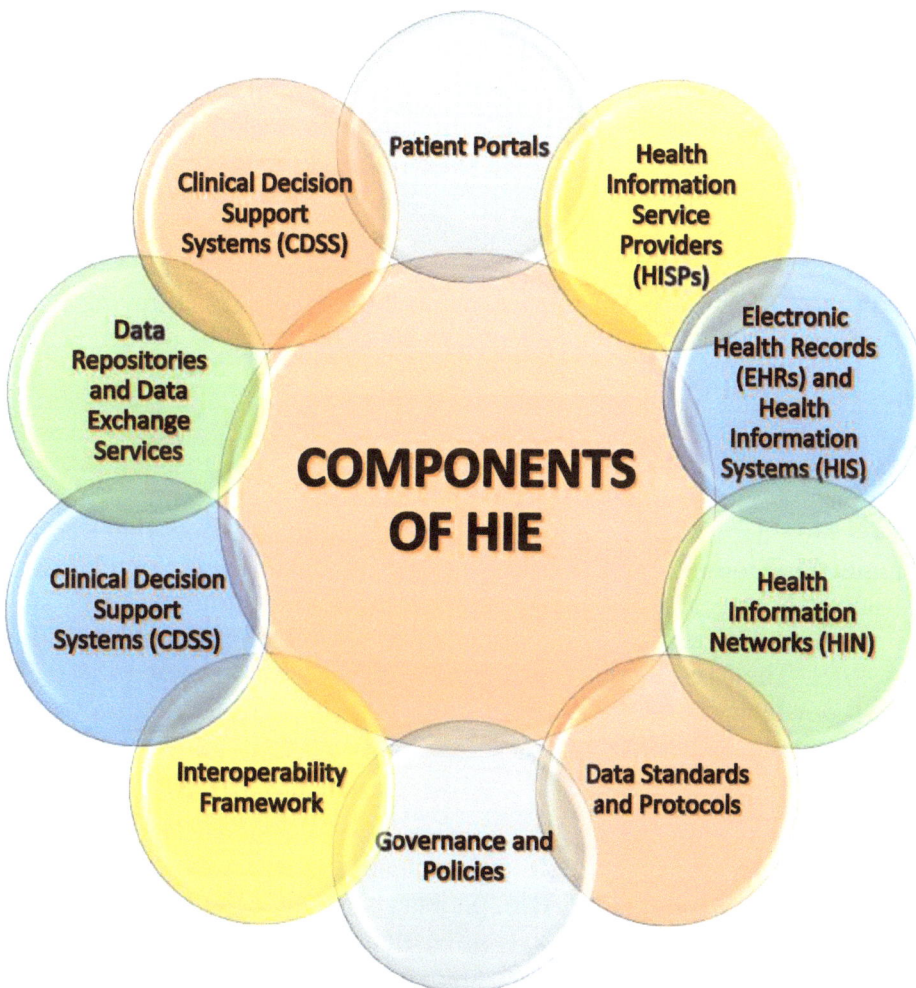

Fig. (2). Components of health information exchange (HIE).

Data Standards and Protocols

At the core, HIE requires a set of data standards and protocols to permit the reliable exchange of health information between different platforms in an operational, understandable manner. HL7 (Health Level Seven) combines with data formats such as CCD (Continuity of Care Document) and FHIR (Fast Healthcare Interoperability Resources) to facilitate the structuring and formatting of diverse types of data across healthcare systems. These protocols specify message format and content, providing a standard means for systems to interpret exchanged data. Standardisation is essential because it makes health IT system communication seamless and secure [36 - 38].

Health Information Networks (HIN)

A health information network (HIN) is an infrastructure that enables the free flow of data between providers, organisations, and systems. These networks are privately or publicly owned and managed according to specific rules, agreements, and protocols to provide security and privacy. The network is a typical stage in which any part of the ecosystem (hospitals, clinics, labs, insurance companies, etc) can share and view patients' data with complete security in real-time. HINs help healthcare organisations achieve system interoperability, allowing for better care coordination and enhancing patient data accessibility when needed [39 - 41].

Health Information Service Providers (HISPs)

Health Information Service Providers (HISPs) are organisations that offer services that support secure health data exchange between the facilities of different healthcare providers. HISPs are provided by third-party vendors that manage the communication, routing, and securing of patient data. They provide technical infrastructure and services with encryption, secure messaging, and data storage. HISPs help guarantee the safe and lawful exchange of information by abiding by privacy laws. Their responsibilities include the help in promoting the technical side of HIE, which operates by configuring the secure messaging protocols and maintaining the infrastructure needed for data exchange [42 - 44].

Patient Portals

Patient portals are safe and secure online spaces where patients can view and control their health information. Also, patients can access their records within the patient portal to view things like lab results, medication lists and other data shared through HIE. Patients are granted transparency and involvement in their healthcare through these gateways. These portals enable patients to access their health data and the potential for better self-management, preventive care, and overall communication between both parties. These portals would allow patients to view their health data, helping them better manage themselves, encouraging preventive care, and improving communication between patients and healthcare providers. Patient portals are imperative for elevating patient engagement and health literacy [45 - 47].

Data Security and Privacy Measures

The essential aspects of HIE are patient data security and privacy. Healthcare data is sensitive, so the security of this information must be ensured, and access to it should be monitored, with strong security mechanisms that prevent unauthorised access and guard against cyberattacks or other forms of data breaches. Encryption, authentication protocols, and firewalls need to be secured, and safe methods for data transmission are a must, along with access control mechanisms. These rules allow for a properly controlled and private way of exchanging patient data, providing trust in the system from the patient's side [48 - 50].

Interoperability Framework

Interoperability is necessary for HIE, enabling different platforms to communicate and share information, even if built on other technologies or standards. Interoperability frameworks consist of the processes and technical specifications that allow systems from different vendors or organisations to work together and seamlessly exchange data. These frameworks provide protocols, data standards, and technical specifications for translating and sharing data currently specialised in different healthcare systems. The provision across-the-board of healthcare providers, payers, and patients to access and share health data also helps in a more connected ecosystem of healthcare [51 - 53].

Clinical Decision Support Systems (CDSS)

HIE networks incorporate Clinical Decision Support Systems (CDSS) to deliver real-time, evidence-based guidance that aids healthcare providers in patient care. CDSS can provide alerts, reminders, and guidelines based on the vast dataset now available through HIE, which includes the patient's medical history and conditions. This assists clinicians in making better decisions, protecting patient security, and averting human medical errors. CDSS can either flag potential drug interactions, recommend screening tests based on a patient's age and risk factors, or inform providers about changes in a patient's condition that require attention [54 - 56].

Data Repositories and Data Exchange Services

Data repositories store and aggregate healthcare data within centralised databases or cloud-based storage systems. HIE network repositories that store patient records and medical data exchanged between healthcare providers. These platforms make it easy for authorised personnel to quickly and securely access patient information, even if the data is distributed across disparate locations. Data exchange services help to transmit this data between healthcare entities so that the correct information can be sent to the right place and at the right time. These services can be cloud-based platforms or shared data hubs, enabling healthcare providers to transmit, receive, and access the information from any other system [57 - 59].

Governance and Policies

Governance and policies are vital to the successful operation of an HIE. These policies establish the rules and regulations for sharing, accessing, and protecting data within the HIE network. Governance structures typically comprise stakeholders such as healthcare providers, policymakers, and legal entities, who work together to ensure that HIE systems adhere to legal and ethical standards. These policies address consent management, access to data, user authentication, ownership of data, and secure information exchange. Governance sustains trust in this system, enables compliance with regulations, and guides the future development of HIE [60 - 62].

BENEFITS OF HIE IN OPTIMIZED HEALTHCARE

Health Information Exchange (HIE) offers numerous critical benefits in optimising healthcare by enhancing efficiency, improving care quality, and reducing costs, which are summarised in Fig. (**3**). Integrating HIE into healthcare systems supports a more interconnected and collaborative environment, benefiting patients, healthcare providers, and the healthcare ecosystem [63]. The key benefits of HIE in optimised healthcare include:

Improved Care Coordination

This is one of the most essential advantages of HIE. HIE provides immediate and accurate access to patient health records, which in turn enables practitioners to make better decisions effectively, maintaining care without breaks and silos in different practices. It is critical, of course, for patients with chronic disease who see several sorts of specialists. HIE helps keep all providers in the loop about a patient's treatment history, medications, and lab results, which reduces fragmented care, miscommunication and conflicting treatments. They allow the continuous transfer of care as patients move between hospitals, outpatient clinics, or any other home care [64 - 66].

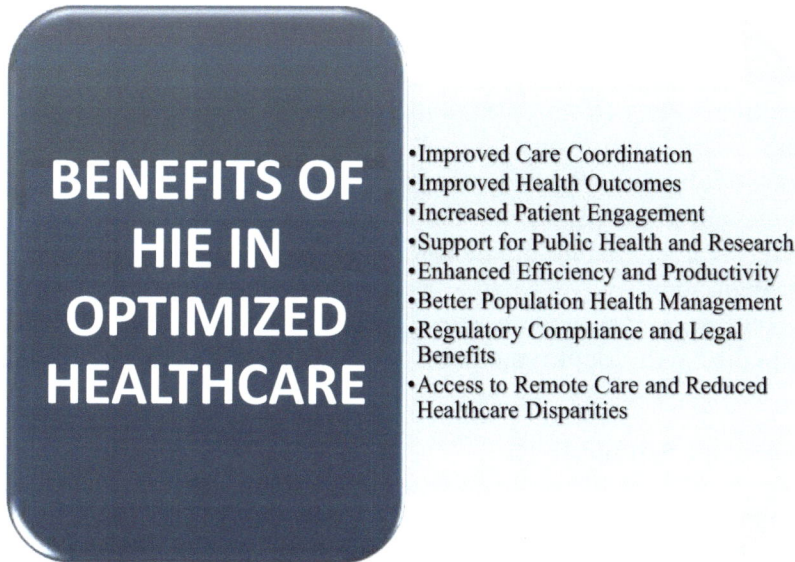

- Improved Care Coordination
- Improved Health Outcomes
- Increased Patient Engagement
- Support for Public Health and Research
- Enhanced Efficiency and Productivity
- Better Population Health Management
- Regulatory Compliance and Legal Benefits
- Access to Remote Care and Reduced Healthcare Disparities

Fig. (3). Benefits of HIE in optimized healthcare.

Improved Health Outcomes

More timely and accurate diagnoses lead to earlier, more effective treatment plans through HIE, which drives down costs while increasing the quality of care. Access to complete and real-time patient data means healthcare providers can act swiftly in urgent situations. HIE can also prevent further chronic condition complications and decrease the progression of these conditions, as HIE allows trends in patient health to be observed over time. Additionally, because HIE prevents unnecessary rounds of testing and procedures, patients are not at risk of the potential harms associated with repeat diagnostics or interventions. This, in turn, yields a more impactful patient journey, better health outcomes, and enhanced public health [67, 68].

Increased Patient Engagement

HIE increases patient engagement by enabling patients to access their health records *via* patient portals or mobile applications. Greater transparency will put patients in charge of their care by providing them with the information they need to understand their medical conditions, treatment choices and progress. While armed with their data, patients can ask better questions, arrange follow-up visits, and comply with medication and treatment regimens. Ensuring the management of patients with chronic conditions, not being re-admitted to hospitals, and falling under preventive care guidelines wouldn't be successful without patient engagement. Patient engagement leads to better patient outcomes [69, 70].

Support for Public Health and Research

HIE aids public health efforts, offering pseudonymised aggregate data for disease surveillance, health trend monitoring and population health tracking. This information will assist public health authorities in identifying outbreaks, tracking chronic disease rates, and planning targeted interventions. The data provided by HIE are also used in research, encouraging clinical studies to develop strategies to provide better treatment, identify risk factors, and evaluate the overall well-being of interventions. Real-time health data can speed up and improve research accuracy while expediting the deployment of new therapies and public health interventions [71, 72].

Enhanced Efficiency and Productivity

HIE minimises healthcare providers' time hunting to access, retrieve and likely request patient information. Integrating patient health care data in a centralised system or network eliminates, to a great extent, administrative burdens and offers channels for streamlining workflows. Healthcare providers can focus more on providing exemplary care and less on paperwork and manual data transfers. In addition, HIE also assists telemedicine and other distance healthcare delivery by allowing physicians to access and extract patient data whenever needed to provide better care wherever the consultation takes place. Therefore, healthcare providers can serve more patients, streamline workflow, and improve workflow efficiency [73, 74].

Better Population Health Management

HIE achieves population health management if it empowers doctors to access a wide array of data on diseases affecting people. This allows patients' information to be analysed and aggregated on trends in health, patient outcomes, and patient populations for better management of these groups. Sometimes, it can identify high-risk populations (*e.g.*, patients with diabetes or cardiovascular diseases) and help decide on early intervention strategies. The proactive approach is used to reduce the prevalence of chronic diseases, enhance preventive care, and maintain the health of entire populations [75, 76]. Fig. (**4**) describes the population health management using HIE.

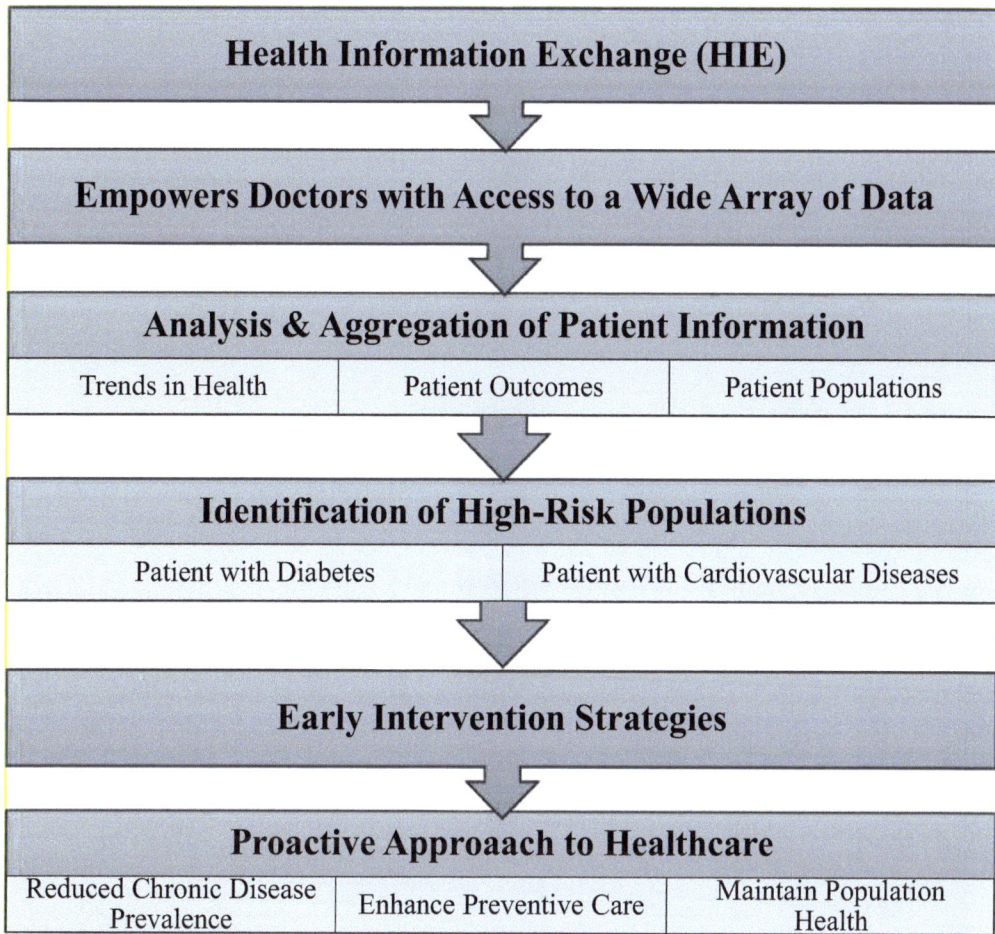

Fig. (4). Flowchart representing population health management through HIE .

Regulatory Compliance and Legal Benefits

HIE is also a way for healthcare providers to stay on top of their legal and regulatory obligations when protecting patient data. HIE uses mechanisms, such as secure data transmission protocols and encryption technologies, to ensure legally compliant patient information exchange through various means, protecting individuals ' privacy issues and preventing unauthorised access. Additionally, HIE monitors sharing activities and provides appropriate access to sensitive health information [77 - 79].

Access to Remote Care and Reduced Healthcare Disparities

HIE helps reduce healthcare access disparities, particularly in rural and underserved areas. Since specialists are not easily found in rural areas, HIE allows patients in remote locations to see a specialist and receive care without travelling long distances. Telehealth services can provide patient consultations, diagnosis, and follow-up care through telephonic, interactive audio-video services that support patient healthcare delivery. This is especially useful for underserved patients due to geographic, financial or logistical challenges. Finally, HIEs help decrease healthcare disparities and eliminate barriers for vulnerable populations to receive care [80 - 82].

CHALLENGES IN THE IMPLEMENTATION

The implementation of HIE systems is fraught with technological, organisational, regulatory, and financial challenges that have limited the adoption and effectiveness of HIE across its key dimensions. Despite this, the interoperability issue continues to be a significant barrier since electronic health record (EHR) systems do not possess standardisation in format and protocols, resulting in discontinuous patient data. And despite the presence of toolboxes like HL7 and FHIR, nonhomogeneous use disrupts communication. Data privacy and security issues create a burden with attacks that necessitate strong encryption and authentication, coupled with compliance obligations diverting staff time. A limited ability to afford the high costs of infrastructure, integration, and staff training is additionally caused by provincial financial constraints, which are common in small practice settings and rural clinics [83, 84].

Even if data is standardised, the need to integrate across different systems adds another layer of complexity, resulting in inaccurate shared information. Healthcare providers' resistance to change due to worries about workflow disruption and lack of trust in shared data points again points to the importance of rigorous training and support requirements. With such additional layers of complexity, many providers struggle to successfully navigate these legal and regulatory barriers, which bind them in diverse ways around data sharing, liability issues with data use, consent management, *etc*. The main issues HIE platforms face are a lack of flexibility with scalability or their inability to handle growing data amounts and new actors spawned by such data. Poor technology infrastructure in underdeveloped areas and inadequate financial incentives hamper adoption [85, 86].

Addressing these challenges will involve a streamlined strategy focusing on standardisation, security, funding, and inclusive policies. Overcoming these hurdles will empower smoother care coordination, improve patient outcomes, and drive economies of scale within health systems by capitalising on the benefits of HIE [87].

LEVERAGING TECHNOLOGY FOR EFFICIENT HIE

HIE seeks to promote high-quality, cost-effective clinical care across all healthcare settings by making available health data where and when it is most needed. Standardised data formats, such as those defined by standards like HL7, CCD, FHIR, *etc.*, and interoperability frameworks facilitate meaningful information exchange between various electronic health record (EHR) systems [88].

A cloud-native infrastructure provides scalable, secure, and accessible central data management services that are cost-effective and cost-effective in real time. With blockchain-enabled, even from an HIE standpoint, we can secure it with distributed and tamper-proof data storage, ensuring transparency while allowing consent *via* smart contracts. It means that these data are cleaned well, reduce duplications, and provide predictive analytics for clinical decision-making; a hub that harnesses the power of artificial intelligence (AI) and machine learning (ML) to deliver high-quality data extraction and optimises the approach to processing data [89].

Telemedicine and home monitoring devices integrated with HIE provide a foundation for continuous data collection and provider access essential to virtual consultations and timely interventions. For example, using advanced data analytics to track trends, such as population health management, includes monitoring disease outbreaks and informing prevention practices. Patient portals put health records in the hands of individuals, and mobile health apps provide the means for people to easily share these records, when necessary, at their discretion, thereby accelerating patient engagement and facilitating whole-patient care [90].

Privacy-preserving technologies such as encryption, secure messaging, and Natural Language Processing (NLP) are significant in securing data at rest, communicating securely, and analysing unstructured formats efficiently. Next, providing the ability to access real-time data in the cloud-based EHR keeps databases in sync and up-to-date for accurate decisions at any time of need, especially in an emergency. Together, these technologies provide a comprehensive HIE ecosystem to drive improved outcomes in care coordination, patient outcomes, and overall operational efficiency [91, 92].

FUTURE OF HIE

HIE is poised for an exciting future, thanks to continuous improvements using technology to provide more streamlined and patient-centred care. Among the most significant trends in the shared health information industry are advances in interoperability, the use of 5G to widen telehealth access, and predictive and preventative healthcare integration [93].

While healthcare systems continue to become better integrated, reaching the ultimate level of interoperability still challenges even the most extensive HIEs. But advances in interoperability are changing that. FHIR is a flexible framework that allows data to be shared more quickly and efficiently while being well-suited for integration with future technologies, like mobile apps and wearable devices. Similarly, new features like Application Programming Interfaces (APIs) are being introduced, allowing developers to create more compatible solutions that work well with existing systems so information can flow easily. Share these innovations are helping to break down data silos and share complete, real-time patient information more effectively [94, 95].

The introduction of 5G technology will be a key component in increasing HIE availability by enabling faster, more responsive, and more comprehensive connectivity throughout health systems. With 5G's faster data transmission speeds, low latency, and greater network capacity over previous technologies, healthcare professionals can now share vast amounts of real-time health data without the same long delays. It will also improve telemedicine services, remote patient monitoring and real-time sharing of diagnostic images and lab results, even in rural or underserved areas where traditional internet access has been impractical. Indeed, 5G will allow healthcare providers to connect and exchange vital patient data in real time from anywhere, making coordinating care easier and providing patients everywhere with coverage for essential medical services [96, 97].

Integrating predictive analytics into HIE platforms transforms healthcare by shifting the focus from reactive to proactive, preventive care. Predictive analytics uses data mining, machine learning, and AI algorithms to analyse large datasets and identify patterns that can predict future health outcomes. By analysing patient history, lifestyle factors, and genetic data, healthcare providers can anticipate potential health risks, such as chronic diseases, before they occur. This allows for early interventions, personalised treatment plans, and better management of chronic conditions, ultimately reducing healthcare costs and improving patient outcomes. Furthermore, predictive analytics within HIE can facilitate population health management by identifying at-risk groups and enabling targeted health interventions to prevent disease onset, promoting a shift toward a more preventative, rather than reactive, approach to healthcare [98, 99].

The horizon for HIE is more about implementing advanced technological advancements to harness shared data, increase healthcare accessibility, and shift towards more predictive and preventative healthcare management. These advances promise more efficiency, greater cost-effectiveness, patient access, and better care management for all patients [100].

CONCLUSION

Health Information Exchange (HIE) are designed to ease the flow of information between healthcare organisations within a country or region to improve patient care, reduce cost and achieve provider objectives; benefits of HIE include improved access to patient's medical records from across different facilities by keeping all necessary data and files at one place. The benefits include better clinical outcomes, care coordination, and patient safety with reduced duplication of tests and procedures. In addition to the problems of siloed healthcare systems, HIE can help bring together all healthcare IT systems and drive efficiencies that will ultimately result in more affordable care delivery. While the potential to drive efficiencies and improvements in health systems is substantial, the continued progress in interoperability, data security, and emergent technologies only accentuates this promise for HIE. A shared dedication to driving HIE forward, enhancing standards and promoting innovation will empower healthcare systems to maximise their potential in the face of current obstacles and a changing landscape for health. Investment in the fundamental technology infrastructure is still required but must also be coupled with more open communications and partnerships. A vision for a future of integrated, frictionless healthcare where patient information flows across borders and care settings underscores the need for continued HIE optimisation efforts. This level of connectivity will not only advance the quality and efficiency of care but guarantee equal access to healthcare services for every population. Through continued partnerships and developments in innovation and technology, the reality of a comprehensive, proactive healthcare system is on the horizon, resulting from improved patient care across the globe.

CONSENT FOR PUBLICATON

All authors have given their consent for publication. The authors authorised Geetika Goel to handle all correspondences.

ACKNOWLEDGEMENTS

Authors are highly thankful to their Universities/Colleges for providing library facilities for the literature survey.

REFERENCES

[1] Hersh WR, Totten AM, Eden K, *et al.* The evidence base for health information exchange. In: Dixon BE, Ed. Health Information Exchange: Navigating and Managing a Network of Health Information Systems. 2nd ed. Cambridge (MA): Academic Press 2023; pp. 213-29. [http://dx.doi.org/10.1016/B978-0-12-803135-3.00014-1]

[2] Holmgren AJ, Esdar M, Hüsers J, Coutinho-Almeida J. Health information exchange: understanding the policy landscape and future of data interoperability. Yearb Med Inform 2023; 32(1): 184-94. [http://dx.doi.org/10.1055/s-0043-1768719] [PMID: 37414031]

[3] Bourquard K, Berler A. In: Health information exchange: The overarching role of integrating the healthcare enterprise (IHE). Introduction to nursing informatics. 2021:101-37.

[4] Rudin RS, Motala A, Goldzweig CL, Shekelle PG. Usage and effect of health information exchange: a systematic review. Ann Intern Med 2014; 161(11): 803-11. [http://dx.doi.org/10.7326/M14-0877] [PMID: 25437408]

[5] Shapiro JS, Mostashari F, Hripcsak G, Soulakis N, Kuperman G. Using health information exchange to improve public health. Am J Public Health 2011; 101(4): 616-23. [http://dx.doi.org/10.2105/AJPH.2008.158980] [PMID: 21330598]

[6] Vest JR. Health information exchange: national and international approaches. Health information technology in the global context. 2012 Jun 25;12:3-24. [http://dx.doi.org/10.1108/S1474-8231(2012)0000012005]

[7] Vest JR. Health information exchange and healthcare utilization. J Med Syst 2009; 33(3): 223-31. [http://dx.doi.org/10.1007/s10916-008-9183-3] [PMID: 19408456]

[8] Nair DP. The Scope and Functions of Health Information Management in e-Health. ECS Trans 2022; 107(1): 9939-55. [http://dx.doi.org/10.1149/10701.9939ecst]

[9] Hettinger KN, Adeoye-Olatunde OA, Russ-Jara AL, Riley EG, Kepley KL, Snyder ME. Preparing community pharmacy teams for health information exchange (HIE). J Ame Pharm Asso 2024 Mar 1; 64(2): 429-36. [http://dx.doi.org/10.1016/j.japh.2023.12.003]

[10] Ben-Assuli O, Shabtai I, Leshno M. The impact of EHR and HIE on reducing avoidable admissions: controlling main differential diagnoses. BMC Med Inform Decis Mak 2013; 13(1): 49. [http://dx.doi.org/10.1186/1472-6947-13-49] [PMID: 23594488]

[11] Tallman EF, Richardson D, Rogow TM, Kendrick DC, Dixon BE. Leveraging HIE to facilitate large-scale data analytics. In: Dixon BE, Ed. Health Information Exchange: Navigating and Managing a Network of Health Information Systems. 2nd ed. Cambridge (MA): Academic Press 2023; pp. 399-421. [http://dx.doi.org/10.1016/B978-0-323-90802-3.00017-4]

[12] Dixon BE. Introduction to health information exchange. In: Dixon BE, Ed. Health Information Exchange: Navigating and Managing a Network of Health Information Systems. 2nd ed. Cambridge (MA): Academic Press 2023; pp. 3-20. [http://dx.doi.org/10.1016/B978-0-323-90802-3.00013-7]

[13] Esmaeilzadeh P, Dharanikota S, Mirzaei T. The role of patient engagement in patient-centric health information exchange (HIE) initiatives: an empirical study in the United States. Inf Technol People 2024; 37(2): 521-52.

[http://dx.doi.org/10.1108/ITP-05-2020-0316]

[14]   West DL. Evaluation of Health Information Exchange Policies in Hospitals Using Electronic Health Records. PhD dissertation. Minneapolis (MN): Walden University; 2024.

[15]   Boden-Albala B. Roadmap for health equity: understanding the importance of community-engaged research. Stroke 2025 Jan; 56(1): 239-50.
[http://dx.doi.org/10.1161/STROKEAHA.124.046958]

[16]   Alsamhi SH, Myrzashova R, Hawbani A, *et al.* Federated learning meets blockchain in decentralized data sharing: Healthcare use case. IEEE Internet of Things J 2024 Feb 19; 11(11): 19602-15.
[http://dx.doi.org/10.1109/JIOT.2024.3367249]

[17]   Cotton KR. Understanding the Current State of Health Information Exchange in Long-Term Care Homes. Master's Thesis. London (ON): The University of Western Ontario (Canada); 2021.

[18]   Esmaeilzadeh P, Sambasivan M. Health Information Exchange (HIE): A literature review, assimilation pattern and a proposed classification for a new policy approach. J Biomed Inform 2016; 64: 74-86.
[http://dx.doi.org/10.1016/j.jbi.2016.09.011] [PMID: 27645322]

[19]   Aldosari B. Patients' safety in the era of EMR/EHR automation. Informatics in Medicine Unlocked 2017; 9: 230-3.
[http://dx.doi.org/10.1016/j.imu.2017.10.001]

[20]   Alotaibi YK, Federico F. The impact of health information technology on patient safety. Saudi Med J 2017; 38(12): 1173-80.
[http://dx.doi.org/10.15537/smj.2017.12.20631] [PMID: 29209664]

[21]   Vest JR, Zhao H, Jaspserson J, Gamm LD, Ohsfeldt RL. Factors motivating and affecting health information exchange usage. J Ame Med Inform Asso. 2011 Mar 1; 18(2): 143-9.

[22]   Gensheimer K, Allard MW, Timme RE, *et al.* Genomic surveillance of foodborne pathogens: advances and obstacles. J Pub Heal Manag Prac 2025 May 1; 31(3): 351-9.
[http://dx.doi.org/10.1097/PHH.0000000000002090]

[23]   Albahri OS, Zaidan AA, Zaidan BB, Hashim M, Albahri AS, Alsalem MA. Real-time remote health-monitoring Systems in a Medical Centre: A review of the provision of healthcare services-based body sensor information, open challenges and methodological aspects. J Med Syst 2018; 42(9): 164.
[http://dx.doi.org/10.1007/s10916-018-1006-6] [PMID: 30043085]

[24]   Orszag PR. Evidence on the costs and benefits of health information technology. In testimony before Congress 2008 Jul 24 (Vol. 24, pp. 1-37).

[25]   Adeniyi AO, Arowoogun JO, Chidi R, Okolo CA, Babawarun O. The impact of electronic health records on patient care and outcomes: A comprehensive review. World J Adv Res Rev 2024 Feb 28; 21(2): 1446-55.
[http://dx.doi.org/10.30574/wjarr.2024.21.2.0592]

[26]   Walker DM. Does participation in health information exchange improve hospital efficiency? Health Care Manage Sci 2018; 21(3): 426-38.
[http://dx.doi.org/10.1007/s10729-017-9396-4] [PMID: 28236178]

[27]   Pawelek J, Baca-Motes K, Pandit JA, Berk BB, Ramos E. The power of patient engagement with electronic health records as research participants. JMIR Med Inform 2022; 10(7): e39145.
[http://dx.doi.org/10.2196/39145] [PMID: 35802410]

[28]   Brands MR, Gouw SC, Beestrum M, Cronin RM, Fijnvandraat K, Badawy SM. Patient-centered digital health records and their effects on health outcomes: systematic review. J Med Internet Res 2022; 24(12): e43086.
[http://dx.doi.org/10.2196/43086] [PMID: 36548034]

[29]   Kouri D. Knowledge exchange strategies for interventions and policy in public health. Evid Policy 2009; 5(1): 71-83.

[http://dx.doi.org/10.1332/174426409X395420]

[30]   Lee C, Burgess G, Kuhn I, Cowan A, Lafortune L. Community exchange and time currencies: a systematic and in-depth thematic review of impact on public health outcomes. Public Health 2020; 180: 117-28.
[http://dx.doi.org/10.1016/j.puhe.2019.11.011] [PMID: 31887608]

[31]   Reeder B, Revere D, Hills RA, Baseman JG, Lober WB. Public health practice within a health information exchange: information needs and barriers to disease surveillance. Online J Public Health Inform 2012; 4(3): ojphi.v4i3.4277.
[http://dx.doi.org/10.5210/ojphi.v4i3.4277] [PMID: 23569649]

[32]   Reeves JJ, Pageler NM, Wick EC, *et al.* The clinical information systems response to the COVID-19 pandemic. Yearb Med Inform 2021; 30(1): 105-25.
[http://dx.doi.org/10.1055/s-0041-1726513] [PMID: 34479384]

[33]   Gao F, Tao L, Huang Y, Shu Z. Management and data sharing of COVID-19 pandemic information. Biopreserv Biobank 2020; 18(6): 570-80.
[http://dx.doi.org/10.1089/bio.2020.0134] [PMID: 33320734]

[34]   Basil NN, Ambe S, Ekhator C, Fonkem E. Health records database and inherent security concerns: A review of the literature. Cureus 2022; 14(10): e30168.
[http://dx.doi.org/10.7759/cureus.30168] [PMID: 36397924]

[35]   Ingolfo S, Siena A, Mylopoulos J, Susi A, Perini A. Arguing regulatory compliance of software requirements. Data Knowl Eng 2013; 87: 279-96.
[http://dx.doi.org/10.1016/j.datak.2012.12.004]

[36]   Holmgren AJ, Adler-Milstein J. Health information exchange in US hospitals: the current landscape and a path to improved information sharing. J Hosp Med 2017; 12(3): 193-8.
[http://dx.doi.org/10.12788/jhm.2704] [PMID: 28272599]

[37]   Feldman SS, Schooley BL, Bhavsar GP. Health information exchange implementation: lessons learned and critical success factors from a case study. JMIR Med Inform 2014; 2(2): e19.
[http://dx.doi.org/10.2196/medinform.3455] [PMID: 25599991]

[38]   Chatterjee A, Pahari N, Prinz A. HL7 FHIR with SNOMED-CT to achieve semantic and structural interoperability in personal health data: a proof-of-concept study. Sensors (Basel) 2022; 22(10): 3756.
[http://dx.doi.org/10.3390/s22103756] [PMID: 35632165]

[39]   Abdulnabi M, Al-Haiqi A, Kiah MLM, Zaidan AA, Zaidan BB, Hussain M. A distributed framework for health information exchange using smartphone technologies. J Biomed Inform 2017; 69: 230-50.
[http://dx.doi.org/10.1016/j.jbi.2017.04.013] [PMID: 28433825]

[40]   Dixon BE, Zafar A, Overhage JM. A Framework for evaluating the costs, effort, and value of nationwide health information exchange. J Am Med Inform Assoc 2010; 17(3): 295-301.
[http://dx.doi.org/10.1136/jamia.2009.000570] [PMID: 20442147]

[41]   Supancik K. Healthcare information exchange. In: Jones S, Groom FM, Eds. Information and Communication Technologies in Healthcare. 1st ed. Boca Raton (FL): Auerbach Publications; 2012; pp. 61-86.
[http://dx.doi.org/10.1201/b11696-5]

[42]   Ajuwon GA, Rhine L. The level of Internet access and ICT training for health information professionals in sub-Saharan Africa. Health Info Libr J 2008; 25(3): 175-85.
[http://dx.doi.org/10.1111/j.1471-1842.2007.00758.x] [PMID: 18796078]

[43]   Gaynor M, Lenert L, Wilson KD, Bradner S. Why common carrier and network neutrality principles apply to the Nationwide Health Information Network (NWHIN). J Am Med Inform Assoc 2014; 21(1): 2-7.
[http://dx.doi.org/10.1136/amiajnl-2013-001719] [PMID: 23837992]

[44]   Igwama GT, Olaboye JA, Maha CC, Ajegbile MD, Abdul S. Integrating electronic health records

systems across borders: Technical challenges and policy solutions. Intel Med Sci Res J 2024; 4(7): 788-96.

[45] Quinn M, Forman J, Harrod M, *et al.* Electronic health records, communication, and data sharing: challenges and opportunities for improving the diagnostic process. Diagnosis (Berl) 2019; 6(3): 241-8.
[http://dx.doi.org/10.1515/dx-2018-0036] [PMID: 30485175]

[46] Onyeaka H, Ajayi KV, Muoghalu C, *et al.* Access to online patient portals among individuals with depression and anxiety. Psychiatry Research Communications 2022; 2(4): 100073.
[http://dx.doi.org/10.1016/j.psycom.2022.100073]

[47] Carini E, Villani L, Pezzullo AM, *et al.* The impact of digital patient portals on health outcomes, system efficiency, and patient attitudes: updated systematic literature review. J Med Internet Res 2021; 23(9): e26189.
[http://dx.doi.org/10.2196/26189] [PMID: 34494966]

[48] Rindfleisch TC. Privacy, information technology, and health care. Commun ACM 1997; 40(8): 92-100.
[http://dx.doi.org/10.1145/257874.257896]

[49] Hiller J, McMullen MS, Chumney WM, Baumer DL. Privacy and security in implementing health information technology (electronic health records): US and EU compared. BUJ Sci & Tech L 2011; 17: 1.

[50] Habeeb Omotunde , Maryam Ahmed . A comprehensive review of security measures in database systems: Assessing authentication, access control, and beyond. Mesopotam J Cybersecur 2023; 2023: 115-33.
[http://dx.doi.org/10.58496/MJCSC/2023/016]

[51] Torab-Miandoab A, Samad-Soltani T, Jodati A, Rezaei-Hachesu P. Interoperability of heterogeneous health information systems: a systematic literature review. BMC Med Inform Decis Mak 2023; 23(1): 18.
[http://dx.doi.org/10.1186/s12911-023-02115-5] [PMID: 36694161]

[52] Ndlovu K, Mars M, Scott RE. Interoperability frameworks linking mHealth applications to electronic record systems. BMC Health Serv Res 2021; 21(1): 459.
[http://dx.doi.org/10.1186/s12913-021-06473-6] [PMID: 33985495]

[53] Panetto H, Zdravkovic M, Jardim-Goncalves R, Romero D, Cecil J, Mezgár I. New perspectives for the future interoperable enterprise systems. Comput Ind 2016; 79: 47-63.
[http://dx.doi.org/10.1016/j.compind.2015.08.001]

[54] Beeler PE, Bates DW, Hug BL. Clinical decision support systems. Swiss Med Wkly 2014; 144: w14073.
[PMID: 25668157]

[55] Chen Z, Liang N, Zhang H, *et al.* Harnessing the power of clinical decision support systems: challenges and opportunities. Open Heart 2023; 10(2): e002432.
[http://dx.doi.org/10.1136/openhrt-2023-002432] [PMID: 38016787]

[56] Lin M, He Y, He P, *et al.* Development and implementation of a clinical decision support system to enhance efficiency and accuracy in medication prescription review in a tertiary care hospital: a retrospective hospital cdss register study. J Multidiscip Healthc 2025; 18: 1043-51.
[http://dx.doi.org/10.2147/JMDH.S505889] [PMID: 40008285]

[57] Yau SS, Yin Y. A privacy-preserving repository for data integration across data sharing services. IEEE Trans Serv Comput 2008; 1(3): 130-40.
[http://dx.doi.org/10.1109/TSC.2008.14]

[58] Savage L, Gaynor M, Adler-Milstein J. Digital health data and information sharing: A new frontier for health care competition. Antitrust Law J 2018; 82: 593.

[59] Esmaeilzadeh P, Mirzaei T. The potential of blockchain technology for health information exchange:

experimental study from patients' perspectives. J Med Internet Res 2019; 21(6): e14184.
[http://dx.doi.org/10.2196/14184] [PMID: 31223119]

[60]   Mamuye AL, Yilma TM, Abdulwahab A, *et al.* Health information exchange policy and standards for digital health systems in africa: A systematic review. PLOS Digital Health 2022; 1(10): e0000118.
[http://dx.doi.org/10.1371/journal.pdig.0000118] [PMID: 36812615]

[61]   Williamson B. Governing methods: policy innovation labs, design and data science in the digital governance of education. J Educ Adm Hist 2015; 47(3): 251-71.
[http://dx.doi.org/10.1080/00220620.2015.1038693]

[62]   Kaushal R, Vest JR, Kierkegaard P. How could health information exchange better meet the needs of care practitioners? Appl Clin Inform 2014; 5(4): 861-77.
[http://dx.doi.org/10.4338/ACI-2014-06-RA-0055] [PMID: 25589903]

[63]   Sun Z, Compeau D, Carter M. Mapping the landscape of health information exchange (HIE) networks in the United States. Comm Assoc Inform Syst 2021; 49(1): 483-514.
[http://dx.doi.org/10.17705/1CAIS.04924]

[64]   Sridhar S, Brennan PF, Wright SJ, Robinson SM. Optimizing financial effects of HIE: a multi-party linear programming approach. J Am Med Inform Assoc 2012; 19(6): 1082-8.
[http://dx.doi.org/10.1136/amiajnl-2011-000606] [PMID: 22733978]

[65]   Myrzashova R, Alsamhi SH, Hawbani A, Curry E, Guizani M, Wei X. Safeguarding patient data-sharing: Blockchain-enabled federated learning in medical diagnostics. IEEE Trans Sust Comp 2024 Jun 4; 10(1): 176-89.
[http://dx.doi.org/10.1109/TSUSC.2024.3409329]

[66]   McCleary NJ, Merle JL, Richardson JE, *et al.* Bridging clinical informatics and implementation science to improve cancer symptom management in ambulatory oncology practices: experiences from the IMPACT consortium. JAMIA open 2024 Oct; 7(3): ooae081.
[http://dx.doi.org/10.1093/jamiaopen/ooae081]

[67]   Thaker NG, Gold D, Kim E, Hong J, Jain A, Royce TJ, Thompson R. The evolving role of physician informaticists in oncology in the era of artificial intelligence. AI in Precision Oncology. 2025 Feb 1; 2(1): 11-5.
[http://dx.doi.org/10.1089/aipo.2024.0047]

[68]   Atasoy H, Demirezen EM, Chen PY. Impacts of patient characteristics and care fragmentation on the value of HIEs. Prod Oper Manag 2021; 30(2): 563-83.
[http://dx.doi.org/10.1111/poms.13281]

[69]   Janakiraman R, Park EM, Demirezen E, Kumar S. The effects of health information exchange access on healthcare quality and efficiency: An empirical investigation. Manage Sci 2023; 69(2): 791-811.
[http://dx.doi.org/10.1287/mnsc.2022.4378]

[70]   Fecher K, McCarthy L, Porreca DE, Yaraghi N. Assessing the benefits of integrating health information exchange services into the medical practices' workflow. Inf Syst Front 2021; 23(3): 599-605.
[http://dx.doi.org/10.1007/s10796-019-09979-x]

[71]   Zhang D, Pee LG, Pan SL, Wang J. Information practices in data analytics for supporting public health surveillance. J Assoc Inform Sci Techn 2024 Jan; 75(1): 79-93.
[http://dx.doi.org/10.1002/asi.24841]

[72]   Diamond CC, Mostashari F, Shirky C. Collecting and sharing data for population health: a new paradigm. Health Aff (Millwood) 2009; 28(2): 454-66.
[http://dx.doi.org/10.1377/hlthaff.28.2.454] [PMID: 19276005]

[73]   Alhashmi SM. Knowledge management, health data, and advanced data analytics to expedite solutions in the healthcare industry. In: Digital Healthcare, Digital Transformation and Citizen Empowerment in Asia-Pacific and Europe for a Healthier Society. Academic Press 2025; pp. 231-247.

[http://dx.doi.org/10.1016/B978-0-443-30168-1.00005-0]

[74]   Zhang X, Saltman R. Impact of electronic health record interoperability on telehealth service outcomes. JMIR Med Inform 2022; 10(1): e31837.
[http://dx.doi.org/10.2196/31837] [PMID: 34890347]

[75]   Menachemi N, Rahurkar S, Harle CA, Vest JR. The benefits of health information exchange: an updated systematic review. J Am Med Inform Assoc 2018; 25(9): 1259-65.
[http://dx.doi.org/10.1093/jamia/ocy035] [PMID: 29718258]

[76]   Kharrazi H, Horrocks D, Weiner J. Use of health information exchanges for value-based care delivery and population health management: a case study of Maryland's Health Information Exchange. In: Dixon BE, Ed. Health Information Exchange: Navigating and Managing a Network of Health Information Systems. 2nd ed. Cambridge (MA): Academic Press 2023; pp. 523–4.
[http://dx.doi.org/10.1016/B978-0-323-90802-3.00011-3]

[77]   Kulynych J, Korn D. The New HIPAA (Health Insurance Portability and Accountability Act of 1996) Medical Privacy Rule. Circulation 2003; 108(8): 912-4.
[http://dx.doi.org/10.1161/01.CIR.0000080642.35380.50] [PMID: 12939240]

[78]   McGraw D. Building public trust in uses of Health Insurance Portability and Accountability Act de-identified data. J Am Med Inform Assoc 2013; 20(1): 29-34.
[http://dx.doi.org/10.1136/amiajnl-2012-000936] [PMID: 22735615]

[79]   Esmaeilzadeh P. Benefits and concerns associated with blockchain-based health information exchange (HIE): a qualitative study from physicians' perspectives. BMC Med Inform Decis Mak 2022; 22(1): 80.
[http://dx.doi.org/10.1186/s12911-022-01815-8] [PMID: 35346176]

[80]   Batool A, Lopez A. Healthcare Access and Regional Connectivity: Bridging the Gap. Journal of Regional Connectivity and Development 2023; 2(2): 260-71.

[81]   Assiri H, Mohammmed A, Alotaibi AM, *et al.* Strategies For Improving Health Administration In Rural And Underserved Areas: Bridging Gaps In Access To Care. Journal of Namibian Studies: History Politics Culture 2020; 28: 142-66.

[82]   Kerketta A, Balasundaram DS. Leveraging AI Tools to Bridge the Healthcare Gap in Rural Areas in India. medRxiv 2024.
[http://dx.doi.org/10.1101/2024.07.30.24311228]

[83]   Yeager VA, Vest JR, Walker DM, Diana ML, Menachemi N. Challenges to conducting health information exchange research and evaluation: reflections and recommendations for examining the value of HIE. EGEMS (Wash DC) 2017; 5(1): 15.
[http://dx.doi.org/10.5334/egems.217] [PMID: 29881735]

[84]   Sherer SA, Meyerhoefer CD, Sheinberg M, Levick D. Integrating commercial ambulatory electronic health records with hospital systems: An evolutionary process. Int J Med Inform 2015; 84(9): 683-93.
[http://dx.doi.org/10.1016/j.ijmedinf.2015.05.010] [PMID: 26045022]

[85]   Attallah N, Gashgari H, Al Muallem Y, *et al.* A literature review on health information exchange (HIE). In: Unifying the Applications and Foundations of Biomedical and Health Informatics 2016; pp. 173-6.
[http://dx.doi.org/10.3233/978-1-61499-664-4-173]

[86]   AbuKhousa E, Mohamed N, Al-Jaroodi J. e-Health cloud: opportunities and challenges. Future Internet 2012; 4(3): 621-45.
[http://dx.doi.org/10.3390/fi4030621]

[87]   Campbell RJ. Change management in health care. Health Care Manag (Frederick) 2008; 27(1): 23-39.
[http://dx.doi.org/10.1097/01.HCM.0000285028.79762.a1] [PMID: 18510142]

[88]   Hughes N, Kalra D. Data standards and platform interoperability. InReal-World Evidence in Medical Product Development Cham: Springer International Publishing; 2023; p. 79–107

[http://dx.doi.org/10.1007/978-3-031-26328-6_6]

[89]   Tyagi AK, Tiwari S. Blockchain-enabled smart healthcare applications in 6G networks. In: Tiyagi AK, Ed. Digital Twin and Blockchain for Smart Cities. Hoboken (NJ): Wiley 2024; pp. 459–94.

[90]   Mutanu L, Gupta K, Gohil J. Leveraging IoT solutions for enhanced health information exchange. Technol Soc 2022; 68: 101882.
[http://dx.doi.org/10.1016/j.techsoc.2022.101882]

[91]   Javaid M, Haleem A, Singh RP, Gupta S. Leveraging lean 4.0 technologies in healthcare: An exploration of its applications. Adv Biomark Sci Technol 2024; 6: 138-51.
[http://dx.doi.org/10.1016/j.abst.2024.08.001]

[92]   Sultan N. Making use of cloud computing for healthcare provision: Opportunities and challenges. Int J Inf Manage 2014; 34(2): 177-84.
[http://dx.doi.org/10.1016/j.ijinfomgt.2013.12.011]

[93]   Sarkar IN. Transforming Health data to actionable information: Recent progress and future opportunities in health information exchange. Yearb Med Inform 2022; 31(1): 203-14.
[http://dx.doi.org/10.1055/s-0042-1742519] [PMID: 36463879]

[94]   Adler-Milstein J, Dixon BE. Future directions in health information exchange. In: Health Information Exchange. San Diego (CA): Academic Press; 2016; pp. 251–64.
[http://dx.doi.org/10.1016/B978-0-12-803135-3.00016-5]

[95]   Santoro M, Vaccari L, Mavridis D, Smith R, Posada M, Gattwinkel D. Web application programming interfaces (APIs): General purpose standards, terms and European Commission initiatives. Eur. Commission, Louxembourg, Louxembourg, UK, Tech. Rep. JRC118082. 2019.

[96]   Pai DR, Rajan B, Chakraborty S. Do EHR and HIE deliver on their promise? Analysis of Pennsylvania acute care hospitals. Int J Prod Econ 2022; 245: 108398.
[http://dx.doi.org/10.1016/j.ijpe.2021.108398]

[97]   West DM. How 5G technology enables the health Internet of Things. Brookings Center for Technology Innovation. 2016 Jul 14;3(1):20.

[98]   Feldman SS, Hikmet N, Modi S, Schooley B. Impact of provider prior use of HIE on system complexity, performance, patient care, quality and system concerns. Inf Syst Front 2022; 24(1): 121-31.
[http://dx.doi.org/10.1007/s10796-020-10064-x] [PMID: 32982572]

[99]   Oluwatoyin Ayo-Farai , Olamide Sodamade , Maduka CP, Okongwu CC, Sodamade O. Data analytics in public health, A USA perspective: A review. World J Adv Res Rev 2023; 20(3): 211-24.
[http://dx.doi.org/10.30574/wjarr.2023.20.3.2462]

[100] Matheny M, Israni ST, Ahmed M, Whicher D. Artificial intelligence in health care: The hope, the hype, the promise, the peril. Washington, DC: National Academy of Medicine. 2019 Dec;10.

CHAPTER 4

Robotics and Automation in Healthcare Processes

Satyabrata Bhanja[1], **Sunita**[2], **Akhil Sharma**[2], **Akanksha Sharma**[2], **Ashish Verma**[3] and **Shaweta Sharma**[4,*]

[1] *RITEE College of Pharmacy, NH-6, Chhatauna, Mandir Hasaud, Raipur, Chhattisgarh 492001, India*

[2] *R.J. College of Pharmacy, Raipur, Gharbara, Tappal, Khair, Uttar Pradesh 202165, India*

[3] *Mangalmay Pharmacy College, Greater Noida, Uttar Pradesh 201306, India*

[4] *School of Medical and Allied Sciences, Galgotias University, Yamuna Expressway, Gautam Buddha Nagar, Uttar Pradesh 201310, India*

Abstract: The fusion of robotics and automation with healthcare advancements has completely transformed medical procedures to make more streamlined healthcare available. In this chapter, we present the disruptive power based on these advanced technologies to tackle the increasing needs of modern healthcare systems. Precision has been achieved in healthcare through robotics (surgical procedures, patient rehabilitation) and automation (diagnostics, caregiving). Automation streamlines the workflow and reduces operational inefficiencies. Key catalysts such as artificial intelligence (AI), the Internet of Medical Things (IoMT), sophisticated sensors, and real-time data processing help to drive these innovations. Through robotics and automation in healthcare, these systems can provide more precision, fewer human errors, and faster interventions, leading to improved patient outcomes. Additionally, these technologies increase healthcare access in rural and underserved areas through mobile robotic units and telemedicine platforms. However, the implementation of robotics and automation is not always easy. Some barriers include sizeable computational power and memory, expensive R&D costs, ethical considerations, data breach risks, and regulatory hurdles. This chapter further explores new trends like autonomous robotic systems and personalised robotic care and their impact on preventive healthcare. This is applied with the help of real-world case studies that portray how successful machine learning implementations have transformed and enhanced efficiency and accessibility. This chapter delivers an extensive view of the importance of robotics and automation in reconfiguring healthcare delivery with a vision to make the system more efficient and more equitable by relying on technology.

Keywords: Artificial intelligence, Advanced sensors, Automation, Data security, Internet of medical things, Real-time data, Robotics.

---
[*] **Corresponding author Shaweta Sharma:** School of Medical and Allied Sciences, Galgotias University, Yamuna Expressway, Gautam Buddha Nagar, Uttar Pradesh 201310, India; E-mail: shawetasharma@galgotiasuniversity.edu.in

INTRODUCTION

The advancement in healthcare technologies has been a game changer, changing how we deliver medical care and thus enabling higher efficiency, immediacy, and patient health outcomes. Primitive instruments like scalpels and forceps, natural remedies, and ancient healing handled the preliminary areas of the big picture, known as modern medicine. Mass-produced surgical instruments, vaccines, and antibiotics have revolutionised how we prevent or treat diseases. By the 1950s, increasingly sophisticated diagnostic and surgical approaches flowed from the introduction of technologies such as X-rays, ultrasound imaging, and, in many cases, a heart-lung machine. Towards the end of the 20th century, we saw the digital revolution with computerised medical records, advanced imaging modalities such as MRIs and CT scans, and robotic-assisted surgery, including the Puma 560 system [1 - 3].

The 21st century has seen the convergence of artificial intelligence (AI), robotics, and the Internet of Medical Things (IoMT) to revolutionise healthcare. Some robotic surgical systems, rehabilitation devices, and caregiving robots now have greater precision and care. At the same time, wearables and telehealth platforms now provide more remote care options and AI-driven analytics, allowing earlier disease identification and personalised treatment. These trends indicate precision medicine, autonomous robotic systems, and further automation of administrative processes, which help alleviate healthcare disparities and achieve better health outcomes. This rapid advancement is a testament to the importance of robotics and automation in making health systems more efficient, patient-centered, and less costly [4 - 6].

Healthcare robotics and automation are a multi-disciplinary field focusing on the theory, design, development, and implementation of robots for healthcare (sometimes called robotic medicine practice) to perform tasks more effectively than humans with precision. Robotics is building and using intelligent machines that can perform complex actions, some types of surgery, and assist in rehab or caregiving with minimal human intervention [7, 8]. Automation simplifies repetitive and labour-intensive tasks by deploying algorithms, software and machinery such as automated diagnostics, pharmacy systems, or administrative workflows. Robotics and automation are a wide array of technologies that span from the clinical domain, including robot-assisted surgeries, to autonomous diagnostics, up to operational domains, such as hospital logistics and telemedicine delivery. These technologies aim to enhance the patient experience, streamline operations and democratise access to healthcare. Integrating robotics and automation via artificial intelligence, machine learning, and the Internet of Medical Things (IoMT) is a fundamental mechanism to shift the paradigm in healthcare delivery processes for scalable, precision-driven, patient-centric care systems [9, 10].

Importance of Robotics and Automation in Modern Healthcare

Robotics and automation play a crucial role in modern healthcare, which is depicted in Fig. (**1**). Examples of these technologies include those that can augment the precision of processes, decrease human errors, and ensure better patient outcomes. Robotic surgical systems, on the other hand, provide unparalleled precision with minimally invasive surgery, leading to faster recovery times and fewer complications. Automation automates routine office work such as diagnostics, laboratory tests, and administrative processes, so medical staff, doctors and administrators have more time to better care for patients [11, 12].

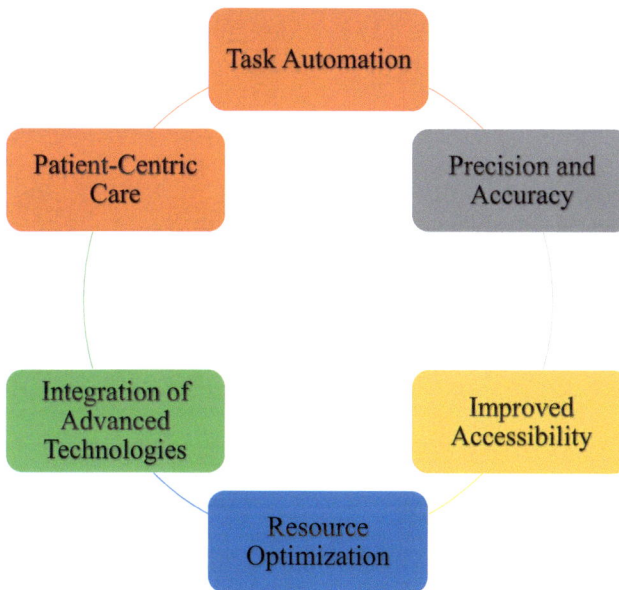

Fig. (1). Importance of robotics and automation in modern healthcare.

Moreover, robotics is an indispensable part of this realm, including specialised tools, and automation greatly enhances accessibility by bringing healthcare to a more significant number of vulnerable populations through telemedicine-enabled robots and mobile diagnostic units embedding machine intelligence. In addition, they improve patient experience and engagement with connected care solutions such as robotic rehabilitation devices and automated drug delivery systems. This technology also optimises the use of resources, reduces operational costs, and eases the pressure on hospital staff [13, 14].

By providing scalable and sustainable solutions, robotic automation technologies play a crucial role in addressing the issue of ageing populations, increasing healthcare costs, and reducing a global shortage of skilled professionals facing our healthcare systems. Incorporating innovative technologies such as AI, the Internet of Medical Things (IoMT), and data analytics, robotics, and automation have evolved beyond essential treatment to foster preventive, diagnostic, and therapeutic innovation. This is not to be underestimated; they are the conduits of change responsible for changing healthcare from an inefficient and exclusive organisation to a patient-focused, easily accessible, and cost-effective [15, 16].

Alignment with Healthcare Efficiency and Accessibility Goals

Robotics and automation align closely with healthcare efficiency and accessibility goals by enhancing healthcare delivery, reducing operational burdens, and ensuring equitable access to care [17]. These technologies optimise healthcare systems in several ways:

Improved Operational Efficiency

Surgery, diagnostics, medication dispensing and filling, and administrative functions benefit from robotics and automation. Surgical robotic systems, through robotics, are a great example. They reduce human intervention, which mitigates errors and produces better outcomes during surgeries in less time. Automated systems in laboratories and pharmacies can accelerate operations such as sample analysis and filling prescription requirements, allowing health professionals to accommodate more cases while taking care of quality [18, 19].

Reduction in Costs

Healthcare organisations can save vast amounts of money by automating tasks that would do the same thing over and over, while enhancing the accuracy of treatments. That is also why automating repetitive tasks in this area gives healthcare professionals their most valuable resource: time to spend more essential and judgement-based decision-making and patient care. In addition, surgeries and rehabilitation systems based on robotics may shorten the recovery time, which is cost-saving due to the reduction of hospitalisation or post-treatment [20, 21].

Enhanced Accessibility

Health care can be expanded through robotics and automation, particularly for the underserved and rural populations. These telemedicine robots provide access to healthcare professionals who can consult and diagnose patients in remote areas, allowing patients to be treated without any geographic or infrastructural obstacles. From automated diagnostic tools to mobile health units, these technologies extend care to rural areas where a medical expert's availability is otherwise far-fetched. Moreover, caregiving and rehabilitation robotic systems have been found to improve care for the elderly and handicapped, giving them more independence with continuous assistance [22, 23].

Personalised and Patient-Centered Care

These personalised healthcare experiences can be facilitated by robotics and automation. AI-driven systems coupled with robotics allow for the analysis of patient records and the delivery of personalised treatment plans. Many robotic rehabilitation devices, such as the one I recently saw in Japan, vary the therapy levels depending on how well a patient is doing, leading to a more efficient recovery. This patient-centred approach consistently offers care that leads to the right treatment therapy that is individualised as per the patient [24, 25].

Applications of Robotics in Healthcare

Robotics has transformed various aspects of healthcare, enhancing precision, efficiency, and patient care. The primary applications are as follows.

Surgical Robotics

Robotic systems have transformed surgical operations, creating opportunities to complete minimally invasive procedures with better accuracy and faster recovery. The da Vinci Surgical System is among the most commonly used robotic devices in urology, gynaecology, and other surgeries. The smaller incisions cause less trauma to the patient and provide greater pre-calibration rate and mechanical coordination during surgical moves, resulting in faster healing speeds and better patient outcomes [26, 27].

Rehabilitation Robotics

This is also among the widening range of application areas in rehabilitation robotics to help patients recover mobility. When people need to relearn how to walk or use their arms after an injury or stroke, robotic devices can help by directing movement and augmenting motor learning. Meanwhile, robotic prosthetics and exoskeletons are offering game-changing solutions for individuals with limb loss or spinal cord injuries, giving them hope for more mobility in their daily lives. They tailor these technologies to each patient, allowing for individualised and improved rehabilitation [28, 29].

Caregiving Robots

Caregiving robots are helping to address the growing need for elderly care and mental health therapy. Robots like Pepper and Paro offer companionship, monitor health metrics, and assist with daily activities, improving the quality of life for elderly patients and promoting their independence. For instance, in mental health, robots supplement therapy by engaging with patients who have autism or social anxiety, providing an interactive and nonjudgmental experience that can lead to higher emotional well-being and therapeutic outcomes [30, 31].

Diagnostic Automation

For instance, in mental health, robots supplement therapy by engaging with patients who have autism or social anxiety, providing an interactive and non-judgmental experience that can lead to higher emotional well-being and therapeutic outcomes [32, 33].

Logistics and Pharmacy Automation

Robotics is improving logistics and how pharmacy operations are conducted more efficiently in healthcare facilities. Robotic medication dispensers fill prescriptions automatically to ensure accuracy and decrease errors in drug delivery. Autonomous mobile robots are also used in hospital logistics to deliver supplies, equipment, and specimens between various departments, freeing up hospital staff from moving all this material so they can concentrate on patient care instead. These digital healthcare practices help make hospital operations more effective and provide better patient service [34, 35].

Technological Enablers

Integrating robotics and automation in healthcare has been made possible by combining advanced technologies that drive innovation, enhance functionality, and enable scalable solutions. These technological enablers are crucial to robotics's widespread adoption and success in healthcare [36]. Some critical enablers are summarised in Fig. (**2**).

Artificial Intelligence (AI) and Machine Learning (ML)

Enhancing Robotic System Capabilities through AI and ML Algorithms, Robots can quickly analyse trends and act instantaneously using AI to process enormous datasets. AI can aid in precision surgical procedures, such as robotic surgery. In diagnostics, AI takes an existing system, medical imaging and pathology slides and analyses them with incredible accuracy, allowing clinicians to maximise early-stage disease detection. Robots can adjust to individual patients thanks to machine learning, which enables the robot to learn from experience and improve with time [37, 38].

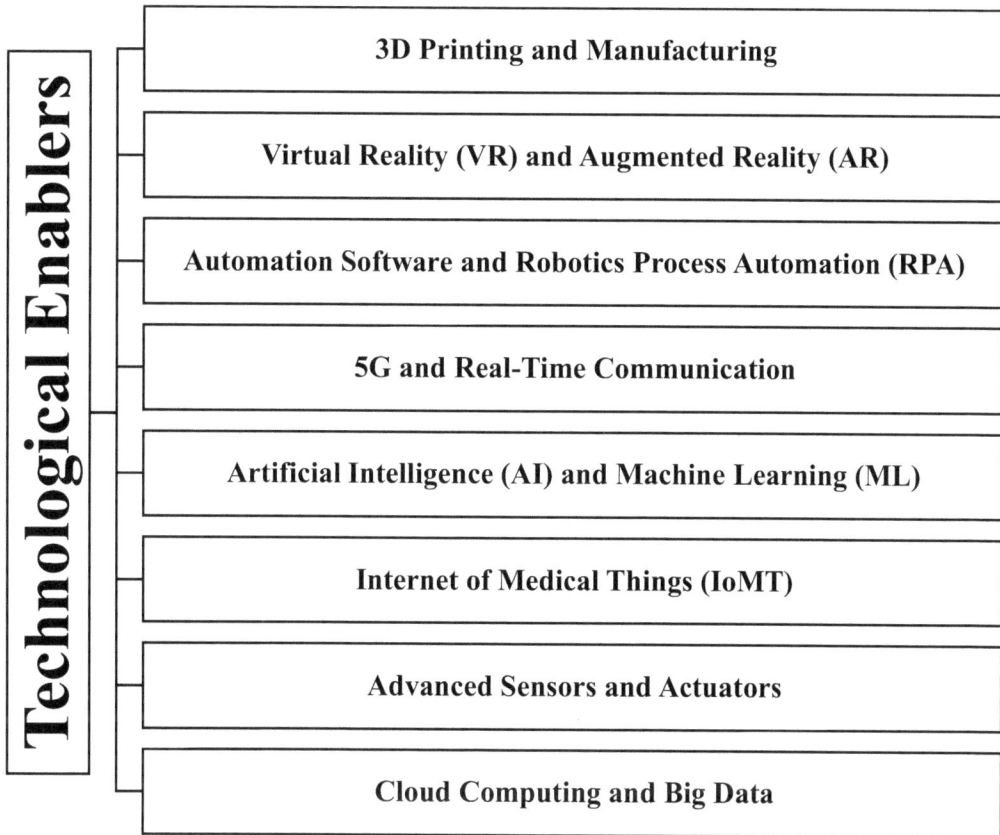

Fig. (2). Technological enablers of robotics and automation in healthcare.

Internet of Medical Things (IoMT)

It includes all connected devices and sensors that relay real-time patient data to healthcare workers. A network of connected devices enables robotic systems that can interact with medical equipment to provide ongoing monitoring and assistance. For instance, robotic surgical systems might one day be able to interact with vital sign monitors. The exoskeleton could monitor patients' movements and tailor therapy based on feedback from what is occurring in real time. Wearables and telemedicine robots, IoMT, also offer remote patient monitoring to ensure continuous care [39, 40].

Advanced Sensors and Actuators

Sensors and actuators are the sensory organs and limbs of robotic systems that ensure accurate motion and the movement and interaction of robots with patients and within medical environments. For example, sensors (pressure or temperature sensors, motion detectors) allow robots to sense their environment and adapt their actions in consequence. Actuators that move robotic limbs or tools provide the precise movement necessary for surgery and therapy. Advanced sensor technology enhances the safety and efficacy of healthcare robots, enabling them to interact with humans safely and efficiently [41, 42].

Cloud Computing and Big Data

Robotic systems and healthcare devices produce a massive amount of data; cloud computing is the backbone to save them so that they can be analysed later. This provides immediate access to patient data, operative notes and diagnostic findings necessary for telesurgery and robotic surgery. Additionally, state-of-the-art data analytics enable the capture and codification of queries, creating the opportunity to improve patient outcomes [43, 44]. Fig. (**3**) highlights the role of cloud computing in healthcare data management and robotic surgery.

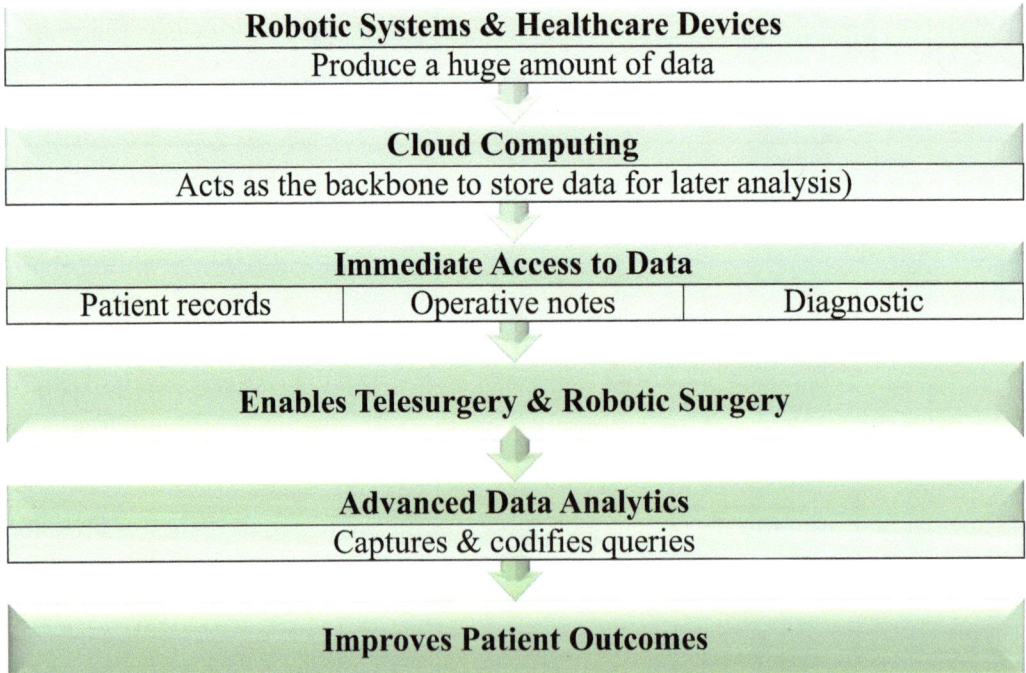

Robotic Systems & Healthcare Devices
Produce a huge amount of data

Cloud Computing
Acts as the backbone to store data for later analysis)

Immediate Access to Data

| Patient records | Operative notes | Diagnostic |

Enables Telesurgery & Robotic Surgery

Advanced Data Analytics
Captures & codifies queries

Improves Patient Outcomes

Fig. (3). Role of cloud computing in robotic surgery and healthcare data management.

3D Printing and Manufacturing

3D printing allows custom robotic devices and prosthetics, too. This will enable it to quickly produce patient-specific instruments, such as implants or robot parts. This increases the accuracy and customisation of healthcare robotics, particularly in rehabilitation robotics, where patient measurements can be used to fashion bespoke exoskeletons or prosthetics. Because of its manufacturing capabilities, 3D printing can produce complicated parts of robots at a relatively low cost and quickly [45, 46].

Virtual Reality (VR) and Augmented Reality (AR)

Robotics incorporating virtual and augmented reality provides surgeons and healthcare workers with improved visualisation tools and training capabilities. AR in robotic surgery overlays key patient data like real-time imaging from the surgeon's point of view, making decision-making easy during surgical operations. VR is being used to train surgeons for robotic-assisted procedures with immersive simulations where they can develop their skills without risking patients [47, 48].

Automation Software and Robotics Process Automation (RPA)

Robotics process automation (RPA) software streamlines provider and payer administrative and operational workflows. Robotic process automation (RPA) can automate appointment scheduling, new patient intake, billing, and inventory management, leading to administrative relief for staff. RPA is used with AI to simplify workflows since it can perform multiple repetitive tasks while maintaining accuracy and uniformity [49, 50].

5G and Real-Time Communication

In healthcare robotics and automation, 5G offers faster real-time communication with ultra-low latency, high data transfer rates, and tremendous network power. This lateral movement empowers remote and telesurgeries where surgeons can direct robotic instruments with unimaginable precision across geographic boundaries, increasing access to specialised care. It is also required to monitor patients in real-time and transfer real-time data from robotic systems and IoMT devices to have timely intervention and provide personalised care. This is especially relevant to surgical and rehabilitative robotics since it allows for a smooth near gigabit communication link from the human operator to precise robotic tools working within the patient and among healthcare teams. 5G will help deliver health care more efficiently, with greater access and quality through the availability of real-time communication between doctors, robotic systems, and their patients [51 - 53].

Impact on Healthcare Efficiency

Robotics and automation have a transformative impact on healthcare efficiency, addressing the growing patient care demands while improving operational processes [54]. Areas where these technologies have a significant influence are shown in Fig. (**4**).

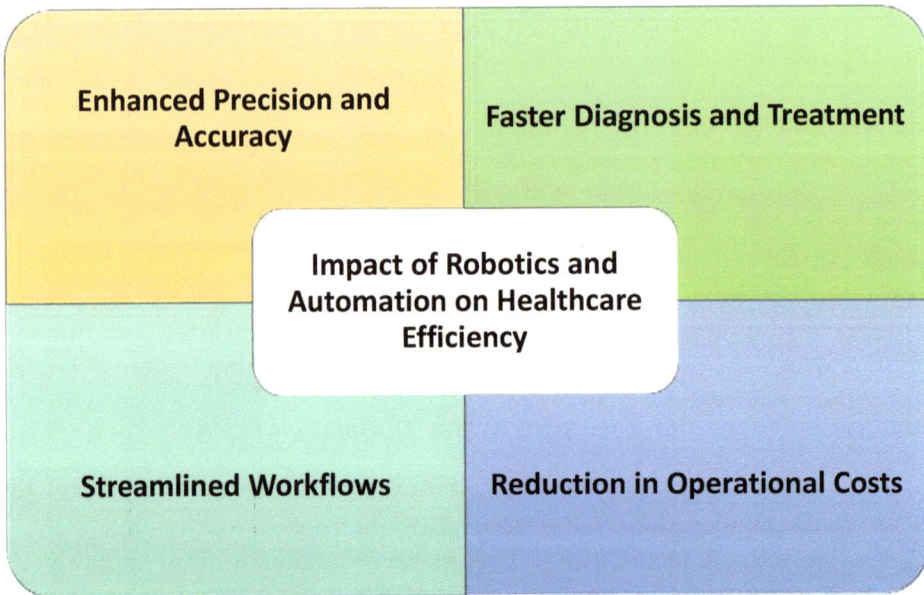

Fig. (4). Impact of robotics and automation on healthcare efficiency.

Reduction in Operational Costs

They optimise the time to perform essential duties and help cut operational costs by facilitating complex tasks and eliminating human errors. Surgery, diagnostics, and medication management automation takes pressure off the manual side of the equation (which can save time and be costly). It decreases the chance of more expensive mistakes. For example, robots can perform surgery with much more accuracy than humans, resulting in fewer complications that lead to costly secondary treatments. Automating administrative functions like billing, appointment scheduling, and patient intake further defrays these costs by reducing process speed and excess staffing [55, 56].

Enhanced Precision and Accuracy

Healthcare interventions with robotics and automation are more precise and accurate. The da Vinci Surgical System translates the movement of a surgeon's hands into robotic instruments that replicate the movements and provide accurate

3D visualisation for complex procedures performed through small incisions, which results in better patient outcomes, fewer complications, and quicker recoveries. Similarly, diagnosis automation (using AI-powered imaging systems) ensures that medical images are analysed correctly, enabling clinicians to make better decisions and reducing diagnostic errors [57, 58].

Streamlined Workflows

Process robotics and automation allow for embedded logic within healthcare, automating repetitive workflow steps. Robots and automated pharmacy machines are better, faster, and less error-prone dispensers of medications; robotic assistants also help with internal logistic flows, transporting supplies within facilities, or supporting transportation between hospital labs to speed up the process. Robotic surgery systems are also used to improve procedure efficiency in operating rooms, decreasing implementation time and moving between operations faster. Administrative automation helps healthcare professionals work more on patient care, thus improving the overall flow of operations [59, 60].

Faster Diagnosis and Treatment

The use of robotics and automation can accelerate the speed of medical processes, thereby enabling quicker diagnosis and treatment. With AI-driven diagnostic tools, the data and images are processed much faster than with a manual approach, wherein they can be used to draw indications of certain diseases in their earliest stages. Diagnostic tools are automated, and lab results can be immediately available for rapid diagnostic processes to ensure timely treatment initiatives. Robotic exoskeletons and prosthetics in rehabilitation help patients to walk or move their joints faster; surgical robotic systems decrease the duration of an operation, necessary for recovery [61, 62].

The flowchart demonstrates how robotics can be seamlessly integrated to speed up medical procedures, from early diagnosis to recovery [63].

Diagnostic tests (such as imaging and lab tests) are performed on the patient.

↓

AI-driven diagnostic tools quickly process data and images.

↓

Automated analysis for the early diagnosis of diseases.

↓

Instant access to lab results for diagnosis.

↓

Making decisions about starting therapy more quickly.

↓

Robotic surgical systems minimise operating time and maximise precision.

↓

Prosthetics and robotic exoskeletons facilitate quicker recuperation.

↓

Better patient recuperation and shorter hospital stays.

Enhancing Accessibility through Automation

Automation and robotics are critical in expanding the reach of healthcare, especially to rural and underserved areas without abundant healthcare resources. As a result, these technologies offer new ways to solve longstanding problems that separate patients from the best care they need and help make sure everyone has access to care [64]. Aspects of enhancing healthcare accessibility through automation include:

Addressing Healthcare Disparities in Rural and Underserved Areas

Health disparities in rural and remote locations can result from a lack of healthcare providers or specialist medical skills. This is where automation and robotics come in: offering access to vital medical care through state-of-the-art telecommunications. Robotic telemedicine systems can enable specialists to provide consultations and surgeries on patients in remote, underserved areas without travelling there. Automating diagnostics, dispensary medications, and patient monitoring helps give the right sort of care consistently and with the best use of these resources, even where they are scarce [65 - 67].

Mobile Robotic Units for Telemedicine

A new generation of mobile robotic units for telemedicine is transforming how healthcare is delivered in remote and rural locations. Each unit is supplied with telepresence robots, diagnostics tools, and AI systems so that health professionals can work away from the patient as they examine, diagnose, and treat them. Alternatively, mobile units are used to visit patients at home who need to travel or move between health centres and prevent journeys to dedicated clinics or hospitalisation. This mobile-first approach to medical treatment makes healthcare available, especially with minimal healthcare infrastructure [68, 69].

Affordable and Scalable Solutions

The use of automation and robotics in health care has its strongest case for scalable, low-cost solutions, one of these technologies' most significant benefits. Automation helps to reduce healthcare costs by decreasing the dependence on highly specialised human labour for diagnostic services, surgery, and patient care. Robotic and automation technologies can be more cost-effective for mass production, reaching a global scale. Further, cloud computing and AI are also much more developed, allowing for easier remote maintenance and updates of these systems, lowering operational costs and making them available to a broad audience [70, 71].

CHALLENGES AND LIMITATIONS

Robotic and automation systems can be game-changing for the healthcare field. Still, several factors must be considered and resolved to allow their widespread impact on healthcare practice. The challenge includes ethical dilemmas, data security, money resource restraints, and other regulatory problems which are summarized in Table **1**.

Table 1. Challenges and limitations of robotic and automation systems in the healthcare field.

Challenge/Limitation	Description
Ethical Concerns and Patient Acceptance	Consumers may not believe as much in robotic-assisted treatments or automated care, asking questions about the merits and ethics of using machines in healthcare. Worries include decreased human interaction, the dehumanisation of care, and concerns about robots' trustworthiness and decision-making ability [72, 73].
Data Security and Privacy	In a world that is becoming increasingly digital, keeping patient data safe from snooping hackers has become a necessity. Automated systems and robotics create reams of data that must be protected from cyber threats, unauthorised access, and breaches of regulations such as HIPAA [74, 75].

(Table 1) cont.....

Challenge/Limitation	Description
High Initial Costs and Resource Constraints	Creating, deploying, and maintaining robotised frameworks and automation innovations are capital-intensive processes. The high initial costs might be a barrier for many healthcare providers, especially in resource-limited settings. Financial constraints should not hinder adoption, particularly among smaller or rural facilities [76, 77].
Regulatory and Legal Barriers	The regulatory frameworks for healthcare robotics are still in their infancy. Issues range from cumbersome approval processes and compliance with safety and quality standards to problems associated with determining liability in case of systems failure or errors. Furthermore, these legal barriers can slow down new technology adoption, making it more difficult for technologies to enter healthcare systems [78].

CASE STUDIES AND SUCCESS STORIES IN HEALTHCARE ROBOTICS AND AUTOMATION

Robotics and automation in healthcare are integrated with great success stories across different applications, such as surgical operations, patient care, and diagnostics. These real-world examples showcase the transformative potential of these technologies, as well as the lessons learned and best practices for their implementation.

Real-World Examples of Successful Robotic Implementations

Da Vinci Surgical System (Minimally Invasive Surgery)

One of the best-known and most widely used robotic surgical systems is the da Vinci Surgical System. It enables surgeons to perform complex operations using tiny incisions instead of traditional open surgery that requires a large cut. The technology has been used for multiple surgeries, including prostate, gynaecological, and cardiac surgery. Hospitals employing da Vinci systems have experienced decreased recovery times, less pain, fewer complications, and shorter hospital patient stays. International adoption of the system has since been successful, as it is ideally suited to more niche applications where accuracy is paramount [79, 80].

Intuitive Surgical's Robotic-Assisted Training Programs

The company that provides the da Vinci system, Intuitive Surgical, has developed extensive robotic-assisted training programs for healthcare providers. The programs simulate actual surgical tasks, allowing surgeons to gain experience in a controlled environment. As a result, surgeons' competency has dramatically increased, and fewer errors occur during robotic surgeries. Hospitals and clinics training staff with these programs have had success stories, reporting much better surgical results and medical staff being more competent than those who did not use virtual reality [81, 82].

Rehabilitation Robotics (ReWalk Exoskeleton)

ReWalk Exoskeleton is the first wearable robotic suit for individuals with spinal cord injuries. This exoskeleton enables users to stand, walk, and climb stairs, greatly enhancing their living standards. The company is currently utilising ReWalk at rehabilitation centres, where it helps patients with mobility impairment become self-sufficient and participate in many activities. ReWalk success stories by patients show the benefits of robotics in rehab and how it can help improve physical function, mental health, and overall quality of life [83, 84].

Robotic Process Automation (RPA) in Hospitals

Hospitals have successfully deployed Robotic Process Automation (RPA) in less demanding administrative tasks such as patient registration, billing, and appointment scheduling. Automation has enabled such systems to perform the same task a hundred times more accurately, leaving well-trained human resources to utilise their potential on more challenging assignments. For instance, RPA at the Cleveland Clinic is one of the key successes that has seen administration costs dramatically drop, higher workflow efficiencies, and far fewer errors in vital processes due to technical bot deployments [85, 86].

Lessons Learned and Best Practices

Comprehensive Training and Education for Healthcare Professionals

A critical component of successful robotic implementations is teaching healthcare professionals to use robotic systems. For example, hospitals that utilised robotic surgical systems like da Vinci noted significant procedure efficiencies and safety benefits due to structured training. Training personnel adequately on robotic systems is crucial for successful implementation [87].

Patient-Centered Approach to Technology Adoption

The success stories remind us that the widespread use of robotics within healthcare means earning patients' trust and ultimate approval. Even when reporting robotic interventions' benefits, risks, and efficacy, it should be transparent with patients. The same goes for robotic surgeries, as patients probably tend to feel more at ease knowing that the procedure would have been extensively discussed and that technology is making it easier to aid their care rather than replacing humans entirely [88, 89].

Collaboration Between Medical and Technical Teams

Another important lesson is the need for close collaboration between medical and technical teams to ensure that robotic systems are successfully integrated into clinical workflows. Many hospitals and healthcare providers, particularly those that have deployed robotic systems successfully, form interdisciplinary teams consisting of engineers and clinicians. This partnership guarantees that the tech meets clinical demands and quality and safety standards [90].

Continuous Monitoring and Upkeep of Robotic Systems

Successful case studies also highlight the importance of ongoing maintenance and system upgrades. Robotics and automation technologies require regular calibration, software updates, and troubleshooting to maintain optimal performance. Healthcare organisations that have established proactive maintenance schedules and support teams experience fewer system failures and ensure uninterrupted patient care [91].

Scalability and Cost-Effectiveness

Many healthcare organisations have learned that robotics and automation must be scalable and cost-effective for them to be sustainable. Institutions that have adopted robotic solutions gradually, starting with smaller pilot programs before scaling up, have found success. Additionally, exploring financing options or partnerships with tech providers has helped manage the high initial costs of robotics and automation [92].

FUTURE TRENDS

The future of robotics and automation in healthcare is marked by exciting developments that promise to revolutionise how healthcare is delivered, making it more personalised, efficient, and accessible. Key emerging trends include advancements in customised healthcare, autonomous systems, integration with wearable devices, and the role of robotics in preventive care. These trends are shaping the future landscape of healthcare and will profoundly impact patient outcomes and system efficiency [93].

Soon, personalised healthcare could become the mainstay of contemporary medical practice, an aspect to which robotics can contribute significantly. As medical interventions transition from "one-size-fits-all" to individualised care plans, robotic systems such as surgical robots, rehabilitation devices and personalised drug delivery systems will be customised to meet a patient's specific needs. Robots will use AI and machine learning algorithms to analyse the fountain of patient data, from genetic traits, environmental information, and lifestyle choices, to craft personalised treatment plans. Robotics can help personalise the robotic-assisted surgeries to each patient's unique anatomy and health status, enhancing accuracy, communications targeting more precise outcomes, and enhanced recovery times [94, 95].

The growth of autonomous robotic systems within the hospital setting will allow personnel to focus on patient care. They will do everything from ferrying supplies and medicines to augmenting surgeries and patient care. They can create their way around the hospital, interact with patients, and aid in the work of medical staff without the need for continuous human oversight. It will increase the throughput of the hospital, reduce human error, and diminish financial turnaround times so physicians can concentrate on direct patient care. Similarly, in addressing staffing deficits, autonomous systems are the solution for automating repetitive and routine tasks [96, 97].

Wearable devices, including smartwatches, sensors, and health trackers, are also continuously being developed and will become key in the future in terms of automation within healthcare. When used with a robotic system, they would allow patients to be monitored continuously for minute-to-minute changes in their health. Wearable sensors can collect data such as heart rate, blood pressure or even blood glucose levels that robots may analyse to spot potential health issues before they become critical. This will enable a new model of care that prioritises prevention and personalised care management for patients with chronic conditions [98, 99].

Using robotics in preventative medicine, we will see a widespread ability to detect and screen symptoms earlier in the disease process and to provide wellness services. With the help of state-of-the-art sensors and diagnostics tools, trained robots would be able to conduct meticulous check-ups and screenings. For example, instead of a human, a robot could perform a batch-processed breast cancer screening or skin cancer detection and assist in evaluating heart disease to catch illnesses further down the line, so treatment would be more impactful. Robots could also be employed in rehabilitation exercises or exercise programs to ensure the preservation of physical health, reduce the onset of diseases, and ultimately minimise hospitalisation [100, 101].

CONCLUSION

The use of robotics and automation to optimise healthcare in terms of efficiency, accuracy and harsh environments shows excellent potential. From the realisation after successful implementations, we have seen that robotic surgery systems, rehabilitation robotics, and AI-driven diagnostic tools enhance patient care while optimising hospital operations. However, questions over morality, expense, and data protection still stand as obstacles to everyday implementation. Looking ahead, the future of robotics in healthcare includes ongoing innovation, advanced integration with wearable devices, and making sure that these technologies can be scaled down and accessible to every healthcare provider. As the healthcare industry adopts this approach, it will be key to focus on building consumer trust, training professionals, and aligning with a regulatory system. The goal to finally enable technology-powered healthcare is only possible through a balanced approach that gifts clinical workflows with automation but is intertwined with human compassion and oversight, opening the doors to an era where healthcare becomes efficient yet genuinely for everyone.

CONSENT FOR PUBLICATON

All authors have given their consent for publication. The authors authorised Dr. Shaweta Sharma to handle all correspondence.

ACKNOWLEDGEMENTS

Authors are highly thankful to their Universities/Colleges for providing library facilities for the literature survey.

REFERENCES

[1]   Yadav S. Transformative frontiers: a comprehensive review of emerging technologies in modern healthcare. Cureus 2024; 16(3): e56538.
        [http://dx.doi.org/10.7759/cureus.56538] [PMID: 38646390]

[2]   Ricketts TC. The changing nature of rural health care. Annu Rev Public Health 2000; 21(1): 639-57.
        [http://dx.doi.org/10.1146/annurev.publhealth.21.1.639] [PMID: 10884968]

[3]   Elendu C. The evolution of ancient healing practices: From shamanism to Hippocratic medicine: A review. Medicine (Baltimore) 2024; 103(28): e39005.
        [http://dx.doi.org/10.1097/MD.0000000000039005] [PMID: 38996102]

[4]   Ghosh A, Chakraborty D, Law A. Artificial intelligence in Internet of things. CAAI Trans Intell Technol 2018; 3(4): 208-18.
        [http://dx.doi.org/10.1049/trit.2018.1008]

[5]   Kyambade M, Namatovu A. Pleasurable emotional states in health-care organizations: the mediation role of employee wellbeing on transformational leadership and job satisfaction. Leadership in Health Services. 2025 Apr 3; 38(2): 299-317.
        [http://dx.doi.org/10.1108/LHS-06-2024-0052]

[6]   Rane N, Choudhary S, Rane J. Towards Autonomous Healthcare: integrating artificial intelligence (AI) for personalized medicine and disease prediction. SSRN 4637894.2023;
        [http://dx.doi.org/10.2139/ssrn.4637894]

[7]   Campesato O. Artificial intelligence, machine learning, and deep learning. Berlin, Boston: Mercury Learning and Information 2020.
        [http://dx.doi.org/10.1515/9781683924654]

[8]   Jakhar D, Kaur I. Artificial intelligence, machine learning and deep learning: definitions and

differences. Clin Exp Dermatol 2020; 45(1): 131-2.
[http://dx.doi.org/10.1111/ced.14029] [PMID: 31233628]

[9] Sultan AS, Elgharib MA, Tavares T, Jessri M, Basile JR. The use of artificial intelligence, machine learning and deep learning in oncologic histopathology. J Oral Pathol Med 2020; 49(9): 849-56.
[http://dx.doi.org/10.1111/jop.13042] [PMID: 32449232]

[10] Oberlin J, Buharin VE, Dehghani H, Kim PCW. Intelligence and autonomy in future robotic surgery. In: Gharagozloo F, Patel VR, Giulianotti PC, Poston R, Gruessner R, Meyer M, Eds. Robotic surgery. Cham: Springer 2021; pp. 183-95.

[11] Jones VA. Artificial intelligence-enabled deepfake technology: The emergence of a new threat Master's thesis. Utica (NY): Utica College 2020.

[12] Gupta G, Raja K, Gupta M, Jan T, Whiteside ST, Prasad M. A comprehensive review of deepfake detection using advanced machine learning and fusion methods. Electronics (Basel) 2023; 13(1): 95.
[http://dx.doi.org/10.3390/electronics13010095]

[13] Deo N, Anjankar A. Artificial intelligence with robotics in healthcare: a narrative review of its viability in India. Cureus 2023; 15(5): e39416.
[http://dx.doi.org/10.7759/cureus.39416] [PMID: 37362504]

[14] Ness S, Xuan TR, Oguntibeju OO. Influence of AI: Robotics in Healthcare. Asian J Res Comp Sci 2024; 17(5): 222-37.
[http://dx.doi.org/10.9734/ajrcos/2024/v17i5451]

[15] Bajwa J, Munir U, Nori A, Williams B. Artificial intelligence in healthcare: transforming the practice of medicine. Future Healthc J 2021; 8(2): e188-94.
[http://dx.doi.org/10.7861/fhj.2021-0095] [PMID: 34286183]

[16] Das SK, Dasgupta RK, Roy SD, Shil D. AI in Indian healthcare: From roadmap to reality. Intelligent Pharmacy. 2024; 2(3): 329-334.

[17] Makar GS, Ratliff J, Albert T, Cheng J, Knightly J. Aligning healthcare systems. In: Ratliff J, Albert T, Cheng J, Knightly J, Eds. Quality Spine Care. Cham: Springer 2019; pp. 273-85.
[http://dx.doi.org/10.1007/978-3-319-97990-8_17]

[18] Reddy K, Gharde P, Tayade H, Patil M, Reddy LS, Surya D. Advancements in robotic surgery: a comprehensive overview of current utilisations and upcoming frontiers. Cureus 2023; 15(12): e50415.
[http://dx.doi.org/10.7759/cureus.50415]

[19] Agrawal A, Soni R, Gupta D, Dubey G. The role of robotics in medical science: Advancements, applications, and future directions. J Auton Intell 2024; 7(3): 1-8.
[http://dx.doi.org/10.32629/jai.v7i3.1008]

[20] McKee M, Correia T. The future of the health professions: navigating shortages, imbalances, and automation. Int J Health Plann Manag 2025 Mar; 40(2): 289-92.
[http://dx.doi.org/10.1002/hpm.3865]

[21] Javaid M, Haleem A, Pratap Singh R, Suman R, Rab S. Significance of machine learning in healthcare: Features, pillars and applications. Int J Intell Netw 2022; 3: 58-73.
[http://dx.doi.org/10.1016/j.ijin.2022.05.002]

[22] Anawade PA, Sharma D, Gahane S. A Comprehensive Review on Exploring the Impact of Telemedicine on Healthcare Accessibility. Cureus 2024; 16(3): e55996.
[http://dx.doi.org/10.7759/cureus.55996] [PMID: 38618307]

[23] Dal Mas F, Piccolo D, Cobianchi L, *et al.* The effects of artificial intelligence, robotics, and industry 4.0 technologies. Insights from the Healthcare sector. In: Proceedings of the First European Conference on the Impact of Artificial Intelligence and Robotics Reading (UK): Academic Conferences and Publishing International Ltd 2019; 88-95.Reading, UK. 2019; pp.

[24] Denecke K, Baudoin CR. A review of artificial intelligence and robotics in transformed health

ecosystems. Front Med (Lausanne) 2022; 9: 795957.
[http://dx.doi.org/10.3389/fmed.2022.795957] [PMID: 35872767]

[25]   Banyai AD, Brişan C. Robotics in Physical Rehabilitation: Systematic Review. Healthcare (Basel) 2024; 12(17): 1720.

[26]   Bogue R. Robots in healthcare. Industrial Robot. Int J 2011; 38(3): 218-23.

[27]   Rivero-Moreno Y, Echevarria S, Vidal-Valderrama C, *et al.* Robotic surgery: a comprehensive review of the literature and current trends. Cureus 2023; 15(7): e42370.
[http://dx.doi.org/10.7759/cureus.42370] [PMID: 37621804]

[28]   Riener R. Rehabilitation robotics. Foundations and Trends® in Robotics. 2013 Dec 29;3(1–2):1-37.

[29]   Díaz I, Gil JJ, Sánchez E. Lower-limb robotic rehabilitation: Literature review and challenges. J Robot 2011; 2011(1): 1-11.
[http://dx.doi.org/10.1155/2011/759764]

[30]   Costanzo M, Smeriglio R, Di Nuovo S. New technologies and assistive robotics for elderly: A review on psychological variables. Arch Gerontol Geriatr Plus. 2024 Jun 25:100056.
[http://dx.doi.org/10.1016/j.aggp.2024.100056]

[31]   Zhao D, Sun X, Shan B, *et al.* Research status of elderly-care robots and safe human-robot interaction methods. Front Neurosci 2023; 17: 1291682.
[http://dx.doi.org/10.3389/fnins.2023.1291682] [PMID: 38099199]

[32]   Habuza T, Navaz AN, Hashim F, *et al.* AI applications in robotics, diagnostic image analysis and precision medicine: Current limitations, future trends, guidelines on CAD systems for medicine. Informatics in Medicine Unlocked 2021; 24: 100596.
[http://dx.doi.org/10.1016/j.imu.2021.100596]

[33]   Maleki Varnosfaderani S, Forouzanfar M. The role of AI in hospitals and clinics: transforming healthcare in the 21st century. Bioengineering (Basel) 2024; 11(4): 337.
[http://dx.doi.org/10.3390/bioengineering11040337] [PMID: 38671759]

[34]   ElLithy MH, Alsamani O, Salah H, Opinion FB, Abdelghani LS. Challenges experienced during pharmacy automation and robotics implementation in JCI accredited hospital in the Arabian Gulf area: FMEA analysis-qualitative approach. Saudi Pharm J 2023; 31(9): 101725.
[http://dx.doi.org/10.1016/j.jsps.2023.101725] [PMID: 37638225]

[35]   Stasevych M, Zvarych V. Innovative robotic technologies and artificial intelligence in pharmacy and medicine: paving the way for the future of health care—a review. Big Data and Cognitive Computing 2023; 7(3): 147.
[http://dx.doi.org/10.3390/bdcc7030147]

[36]   Aggarwal S, Gupta D, Saini S. A literature survey on robotics in healthcare. In 2019 4th International Conference on Information Systems and Computer Networks (ISCON) 2019 Nov 21 (pp. 55-58). IEEE.
[http://dx.doi.org/10.1109/ISCON47742.2019.9036253]

[37]   Knudsen JE, Ghaffar U, Ma R, Hung AJ. Clinical applications of artificial intelligence in robotic surgery. J Robot Surg 2024; 18(1): 102.
[http://dx.doi.org/10.1007/s11701-024-01867-0] [PMID: 38427094]

[38]   Campesato O. Artificial Intelligence, Machine Learning, and Deep Learning. Berlin, Boston: Mercury Learning and Information; 2020.
[http://dx.doi.org/10.1515/9781683924654]

[39]   Srivastava J, Routray S, Ahmad S, Waris MM. Internet of Medical Things (IoMT)-Based Smart Healthcare System: Trends and Progress. Comput Intell Neurosci 2022; 2022(1): 1-17.
[http://dx.doi.org/10.1155/2022/7218113] [PMID: 35880061]

[40]   Dwivedi R, Mehrotra D, Chandra S. Potential of Internet of Medical Things (IoMT) applications in

building a smart healthcare system: A systematic review. J Oral Biol Craniofac Res 2022; 12(2): 302-18.
[http://dx.doi.org/10.1016/j.jobcr.2021.11.010] [PMID: 34926140]

[41]   Zhou S, Li Y, Wang Q, Liu Z. Integrated Actuation and Sensing: Toward Intelligent Soft Robots. Cyborg and Bionic Systems. 2024 Apr 18;5:0105.

[42]   Kalsoom T, Ramzan N, Ahmed S, Ur-Rehman M. Advances in sensor technologies in the era of smart factory and industry 4.0. Sensors (Basel) 2020; 20(23): 6783.
[http://dx.doi.org/10.3390/s20236783] [PMID: 33261021]

[43]   Rajabion L, Shaltooki AA, Taghikhah M, Ghasemi A, Badfar A. Healthcare big data processing mechanisms: The role of cloud computing. Int J Inf Manage 2019; 49: 271-89.
[http://dx.doi.org/10.1016/j.ijinfomgt.2019.05.017]

[44]   Alexandru A, Alexandru C, Coardos D, Tudora E. Healthcare, big data and cloud computing. WSEAS Trans Comp Res 2016; 4: 123-31.

[45]   Wu Y, Liu J, Kang L, *et al.* An overview of 3D printed metal implants in orthopaedic applications: Present and future perspectives. Heliyon 2023; 9(7): e17718.

[46]   Alzoubi L, Aljabali AAA, Tambuwala MM. Empowering precision medicine: the impact of 3D printing on personalised therapeutic. AAPS PharmSciTech 2023; 24(8): 228.
[http://dx.doi.org/10.1208/s12249-023-02682-w] [PMID: 37964180]

[47]   Al-Ansi AM, Jaboob M, Garad A, Al-Ansi A. Analyzing augmented reality (AR) and virtual reality (VR) recent development in education. Social Sciences & Humanities Open 2023; 8(1): 100532.
[http://dx.doi.org/10.1016/j.ssaho.2023.100532]

[48]   Jung T, tom Dieck MC, Eds. Augmented reality and virtual reality: empowering human, place and business. Cham: Springer 2018.
[http://dx.doi.org/10.1007/978-3-319-64027-3]

[49]   Wetsiri W, Paireekreng W. Automating community pharmacy workflows: the impact of RPA on operational efficiency and patient care. J Mobile Multimedia. 2025 Jan; 21(1): 113-47.
[http://dx.doi.org/10.13052/jmm1550-4646.2115]

[50]   Devapatla H, Katti SR. Streamlining administrative processes in healthcare through robotic process automation: a comprehensive examination of RPA's impact on billing, scheduling, and claims processing. Afr J Artif Intell Sustain Dev 2023; 3(2): 14-27.

[51]   Devi DH, Duraisamy K, Armghan A, *et al.* 5g technology in healthcare and wearable devices: A review. Sensors (Basel) 2023; 23(5): 2519.
[http://dx.doi.org/10.3390/s23052519] [PMID: 36904721]

[52]   Kumar A, Nanthaamornphong A, Selvi R, *et al.* Evaluation of 5G techniques affecting the deployment of smart hospital infrastructure: Understanding 5G, AI and IoT role in smart hospital. Alex Eng J 2023; 83: 335-54.
[http://dx.doi.org/10.1016/j.aej.2023.10.065]

[53]   Latif S, Qadir J, Farooq S, Imran M. How 5G wireless (and concomitant technologies) will revolutionise healthcare? Future Internet 2017; 9(4): 93.
[http://dx.doi.org/10.3390/fi9040093]

[54]   Silvera-Tawil D. Robotics in Healthcare: A Survey. SN Computer Science 2024; 5(1): 189.
[http://dx.doi.org/10.1007/s42979-023-02551-0]

[55]   Nimkar P, Kanyal D, Sabale SR. Increasing Trends of Artificial Intelligence With Robotic Process Automation in Health Care: A Narrative Review. Cureus 2024; 16(9): e69680.
[http://dx.doi.org/10.7759/cureus.69680] [PMID: 39429258]

[56]   Ikpe AE , Ohwoekevwo JU , Ekanem II II. Overview of the role of medical robotics in day-to-day healthcare services: A paradigm shift in clinical operations. Ibom Medical Journal 2024; 17(2): 192-

203.
[http://dx.doi.org/10.61386/imj.v7i2.422]

[57]   Iftikhar M, Saqib M, Zareen M, Mumtaz H. Artificial intelligence: revolutionizing robotic surgery: review. Ann Med Surg (Lond) 2024; 86(9): 5401-9.
[http://dx.doi.org/10.1097/MS9.0000000000002426] [PMID: 39238994]

[58]   Vaghani BM. Robotic systems for minimally invasive surgery: enhancing precision, safety, and real-time feedback through industry 4.0 and 5.0. Clinic Med Heal Res J 2025 Aug 19; 5(4): 1368-81.
[http://dx.doi.org/10.18535/cmhrj.v5i04.503]

[59]   Zayas-Cabán T, Haque SN, Kemper N. Identifying opportunities for workflow automation in health care: lessons learned from other industries. Appl Clin Inform 2021; 12(3): 686-97.
[http://dx.doi.org/10.1055/s-0041-1731744] [PMID: 34320683]

[60]   Rothstein DH, Raval MV. Operating room efficiency. In: Raval MV, Rothstein DH, Eds. Seminars in pediatric surgery. Philadelphia (PA): Elsevier 2024; pp. 79-85.
[http://dx.doi.org/10.1053/j.sempedsurg.2018.02.004]

[61]   Kumar Y, Koul A, Singla R, Ijaz MF. Artificial intelligence in disease diagnosis: a systematic literature review, synthesising framework and future research agenda. J Amb Intel Human Comp. 2023 Jul; 14(7): 8459-86.
[http://dx.doi.org/10.1007/s12652-021-03612-z]

[62]   Bissonnette L, Bergeron MG. Diagnosing infections—current and anticipated technologies for point-of-care diagnostics and home-based testing. Clin Microbiol Infect 2010; 16(8): 1044-53.
[http://dx.doi.org/10.1111/j.1469-0691.2010.03282.x] [PMID: 20670286]

[63]   El-Bouzaidi YE, Abdoun O. Advances in artificial intelligence for accurate and timely diagnosis of COVID-19: A comprehensive review of medical imaging analysis. Scientific African. 2023; 22: e01961.

[64]   Vieritz H, Yazdi F, Jazdi N, Schilberg D, Jeschke S, Göhner P. Discussions on accessibility in industrial automation systems. In: 2011 IEEE 9th International Symposium on Applied Machine Intelligence and Informatics (SAMI) Smolenice, Slovakia. New York: IEEE 2011; pp. 111-116.
[http://dx.doi.org/10.1109/SAMI.2011.5738859]

[65]   Samuel-Okon AD, Abejide OO. Bridging the digital divide: Exploring the role of artificial intelligence and automation in enhancing connectivity in developing nations. J Eng Res Rep 2024; 26(6): 165-77.
[http://dx.doi.org/10.9734/jerr/2024/v26i61170]

[66]   Cimolino G, Askari S, Graham TCN. The role of partial automation in increasing the accessibility of digital games. In: Gerling K, Mekler E, Mandryk R, Eds. Proceedings of the ACM on Human-Computer Interaction. New York, USA: Association for Computing Machinery 2024; pp. 1-30.
[http://dx.doi.org/10.1145/3474693]

[67]   Seixas Pereira L, Guerreiro J, Rodrigues A, Guerreiro T, Duarte C. From Automation to User Empowerment: Investigating the Role of a Semi-automatic Tool in Social Media Accessibility. ACM Trans Access Comput 2024; 17(3): 1-25.
[http://dx.doi.org/10.1145/3647643]

[68]   Thinh NT, Hai NDX. Telemedicine mobile robot-robots to assist in remote medical. Int J Mech Eng Robot Res 2021; 10(6): 337-42.
[http://dx.doi.org/10.18178/ijmerr.10.6.337-342]

[69]   Alenoghena CO, Ohize HO, Adejo AO, *et al.* Telemedicine: A survey of telecommunication technologies, developments, and challenges. J Sens Actuator Net 2023; 12(2): 20.
[http://dx.doi.org/10.3390/jsan12020020]

[70]   Husnain A. Smarter Healthcare: harnessing AI for faster, more accurate, and accessible medicine. Global trends in science and technology. 2025 Apr 25; 1(2): 1-22.
[http://dx.doi.org/10.70445/gtst.1.2.2025.1-22]

[71]   Sharma R, Singh D, Gaur P, Joshi D. Intelligent automated drug administration and therapy: future of healthcare. Drug Deliv Transl Res 2021; 11(5): 1878-902.
[http://dx.doi.org/10.1007/s13346-020-00876-4] [PMID: 33447941]

[72]   Mennella C, Maniscalco U, De Pietro G, Esposito M. Ethical and regulatory challenges of AI technologies in healthcare: A narrative review. Heliyon 2024; 10(4): e26297.
[http://dx.doi.org/10.1016/j.heliyon.2024.e26297] [PMID: 38384518]

[73]   Petersson L, Larsson I, Nygren JM, *et al.* Challenges to implementing artificial intelligence in healthcare: a qualitative interview study with healthcare leaders in Sweden. BMC Health Serv Res 2022; 22(1): 850.
[http://dx.doi.org/10.1186/s12913-022-08215-8] [PMID: 35778736]

[74]   Olawade DB, David-Olawade AC, Wada OZ, Asaolu AJ, Adereni T, Ling J. Artificial intelligence in healthcare delivery: Prospects and pitfalls. Journal of Medicine, Surgery, and Public Health. 2024 Apr 16:100108.

[75]   Leenes R, Palmerini E, Koops BJ, Bertolini A, Salvini P, Lucivero F. Regulatory challenges of robotics: some guidelines for addressing legal and ethical issues. Law Innov Technol 2017; 9(1): 1-44.
[http://dx.doi.org/10.1080/17579961.2017.1304921]

[76]   Liu S, Liu G, Zhu B, Luo Y, Wu L, Wang R. Balancing innovation and privacy: data security strategies in natural language processing applications. arXiv preprint arXiv:2410.08553. 2024 Oct 11.
[http://dx.doi.org/10.1109/ICMLCA63499.2024.10754062]

[77]   Eskandar K. Artificial intelligence in healthcare: explore the applications of AI in various medical domains, such as medical imaging, diagnosis, drug discovery, and patient care. Series Med Sci 2023; 4(1): 37-52.

[78]   Islam MR, Ahmed MU, Barua S, Begum S. A systematic review of explainable artificial intelligence in different application domains and tasks. Appl Sci (Basel) 2022; 12(3): 1353.
[http://dx.doi.org/10.3390/app12031353]

[79]   DiMaio S, Hanuschik M, Kreaden U. The da Vinci surgical system. In: Rosen J, Hannaford B, Satava R, Eds. Surgical robotics. Boston (MA): Springer 2011; pp. 199-217.
[http://dx.doi.org/10.1007/978-1-4419-1126-1_9]

[80]   Høyland SA, Holte KA, Gjerstad B, Teig IL. A System Perspective on Implementation and Usage of the Da Vinci Technology at a Large Norwegian Regional Hospital'. SAGE Open 2023; 13(3): 21582440231199315.
[http://dx.doi.org/10.1177/21582440231199315]

[81]   Palep J. Robotic assisted minimally invasive surgery. J Minim Access Surg 2009; 5(1): 1-7.
[http://dx.doi.org/10.4103/0972-9941.51313] [PMID: 19547687]

[82]   Shahrezaei A, Sohani M, Taherkhani S, Zarghami SY. The impact of surgical simulation and training technologies on general surgery education. BMC Med Educ 2024; 24(1): 1297.
[http://dx.doi.org/10.1186/s12909-024-06299-w] [PMID: 39538209]

[83]   Luebbe BN, Woo R, Wolf SA, Irish MS. Robotically assisted minimally invasive surgery in a pediatric population: initial experience, technical considerations, and description of the da Vinci® Surgical System. Pediatr Endosurg Innov Tech 2003; 7(4): 385-402.
[http://dx.doi.org/10.1089/109264103322614268]

[84]   Fukui R, Lovegreen W. Robotics in rehabilitation medicine: prosthetics, exoskeletons, all else in rehabilitation medicine. In: Murphy DP, Ed. Robotics in physical medicine and rehabilitation. Amsterdam: Elsevier 2025; pp. 65–91.

[85]   DiMaio S, Hanuschik M, Kreaden U. The da Vinci surgical system. Surgical robotics: systems applications and visions. 2011:199-217.
[http://dx.doi.org/10.1007/978-1-4419-1126-1_9]

[86]   Nayak A, Satpathy I, Patnaik BC, Gujrati R, Uygun H. Simplified hospital management system: robotic process automation (RPA) to rescue. In: Khang A, Rana G, Tailor RK, Abdullayev V, Eds. Data-centric AI solutions and emerging technologies in the healthcare ecosystem. CRC Press 2024; pp. 281–302.

[87]   Ashrafian H, Clancy O, Grover V, Darzi A. The evolution of robotic surgery: surgical and anaesthetic aspects. Br J Anaesth 2017; 119 (Suppl. 1): i72-84.
[http://dx.doi.org/10.1093/bja/aex383] [PMID: 29161400]

[88]   Beane M. Shadow learning: Building robotic surgical skill when approved means fail. Adm Sci Q 2019; 64(1): 87-123.
[http://dx.doi.org/10.1177/0001839217751692]

[89]   Alaiad A, Zhou L. The determinants of home healthcare robots adoption: An empirical investigation. Int J Med Inform 2014; 83(11): 825-40.
[http://dx.doi.org/10.1016/j.ijmedinf.2014.07.003] [PMID: 25132284]

[90]   Zemmar A, Lozano AM, Nelson BJ. The rise of robots in surgical environments during COVID-19. Nat Mach Intell 2020; 2(10): 566-72.
[http://dx.doi.org/10.1038/s42256-020-00238-2]

[91]   Azadi S, Green IC, Arnold A, Truong M, Potts J, Martino MA. Robotic surgery: the impact of simulation and other innovative platforms on performance and training. J Mini Inva Gyneco 2021; 28(3): 490-95.
[http://dx.doi.org/10.1016/j.jmig.2020.12.001]

[92]   Chitwood WR Jr, Nifong LW, Chapman WHH, *et al.* Robotic surgical training in an academic institution. Ann Surg 2001; 234(4): 475-86.
[http://dx.doi.org/10.1097/00000658-200110000-00007] [PMID: 11573041]

[93]   T MK, B P, Nunavath RS, Nagappan K. Future of pharmaceutical industry: role of artificial intelligence, automation and robotics. J Pharmacol Pharmacother 2024; 15(2): 142–152.

[94]   Khan A, Anwar Y. Robots in healthcare: a survey. In: Arai K, Kapoor S, Eds. Advances in Computer Vision: Proceedings of the 2019 Computer Vision Conference (CVC). Las Vegas (US): Springer Verlag 2020; pp. 280–292.

[95]   Banbhrani SK, Akhter MN, Noureen F, Talpur MS. How AI is revolutionizing healthcare: from personalized medicine and diagnostic tools to drug discovery and robot-assisted surgery. Social Sci Rev Arch 2025; 3(1): 2693–709.

[96]   Chibani A, Amirat Y, Mohammed S, Matson E, Hagita N, Barreto M. Ubiquitous robotics: Recent challenges and future trends. Robot Auton Syst 2013; 61(11): 1162-72.
[http://dx.doi.org/10.1016/j.robot.2013.04.003]

[97]   Graban M. Lean hospitals: improving quality, patient safety, and employee engagement. 3rd ed. Boca Raton (FL): Productivity Press; 2018 Oct 8.
[http://dx.doi.org/10.4324/9781315380827]

[98]   Bacha A, Zainab H. AI for remote patient monitoring: enabling continuous healthcare outside the hospital. Glob J Comput Sci Artif Intel 2025 Jan 23; 1(1): 1-6.
[http://dx.doi.org/10.70445/gjcsai.1.1.2025.1-16]

[99]   Virginia Anikwe C, Friday Nweke H, Chukwu Ikegwu A, *et al.* Mobile and wearable sensors for data-driven health monitoring system: State-of-the-art and future prospect. Expert Syst Appl 2022; 202: 117362.
[http://dx.doi.org/10.1016/j.eswa.2022.117362]

[100]   Yakub F, Md Khudzari AZ, Mori Y. Recent trends for practical rehabilitation robotics, current challenges and the future. Int J Rehabil Res 2014; 37(1): 9-21.
[http://dx.doi.org/10.1097/MRR.0000000000000035] [PMID: 24126254]

[101]   Nesvet JC. Giant magnetoresistive nanosensor analysis of circulating tumor DNA for therapy response monitoring and early detection of cancer. PhD dissertation. Stanford (CA): Stanford University 2020.

CHAPTER 5

Telehealth for Rural and Underserved Communities

P. Syamjith[1], Shaweta Sharma[2], Akanksha Sharma[3], Akhil Sharma[3] and **Mohammad Mansoor[1,*]**

[1] *Devaki Amma Memorial College of Pharmacy, Chelembra, Mallapuram, Kerala 673634, India*

[2] *School of Medical and Allied Sciences, Galgotias University, Yamuna Expressway, Gautam Buddha Nagar, Uttar Pradesh 201310, India*

[3] *R. J. College of Pharmacy, Raipur, Gharbara, Tappal, Khair, Uttar Pradesh 202165, India*

Abstract: Telemedicine has become a life-changing system that changes the medical delivery to rural and other poor localities, improving health status and optimising accessibility, practicality and outcomes. Telehealth acts as a bridge in these areas, offering remote consultations, chronic disease management, mental health services, and educational resources to overcome the geographic and financial barriers to care for those with limited healthcare infrastructure, or rural populations, allowing healthcare to be more widely accessible and less costly while maximising the quality of care. The chapter discusses telehealth's advantages, including linking patients with general practitioners and specialists, saving travel time and cost, and allowing real-time diagnostics. It further highlights the challenges in telehealth implementation, including infrastructure and connectivity problems, digital skills, regulatory obstacles, and resistance. Also, case studies from countries such as Australia, Canada, and India demonstrate successful models of telehealth adoption, and they provide valuable lessons for scaling telehealth in rural contexts. Looking forward, the chapter highlights future opportunities for telehealth initiatives. It suggests integrating emerging technologies such as blockchain and Internet-of-Things (IoT) sustainability policies for governments, followed by sustainable strategies. It concludes by stressing the importance of stakeholder collaboration to ensure that telehealth becomes an enduring solution for healthcare optimisation, ultimately improving health outcomes in underserved communities and reducing healthcare disparities across rural populations.

Keywords: Accessibility, Chronic disease management, Emerging technologies, Healthcare delivery, Optimisation, Rural communities, Telehealth.

---

* **Corresponding author Mohammad Mansoor:** Devaki Amma Memorial College of Pharmacy, Chelembra, Mallapuram, Kerala 673634, India; E-mail: professormmr@gmail.com

INTRODUCTION

Telehealth delivers healthcare services through digital communication technologies, including video calls, phone consultations, and online platforms. This can range from virtual consultations with doctors to remote monitoring of chronic diseases and mental health support. Telehealth is crucial because it breaks down the barriers of geographic separation, limited healthcare professional access, and expensive health costs, especially in rural and underserved regions. Telehealth allows patients to receive care in the comfort of their homes, increasing convenience, reducing travel and wait times, and accelerating medical treatment delivery. Indeed, it has emerged as an integral tool for broadened healthcare access, streamlined healthcare delivery, and redressed inequities in health service delivery, becoming a cornerstone of contemporary healthcare infrastructures [1 - 3].

Telehealth uses communication media, which consist of video-conferencing, mobile applications, wearable devices, and electronic health records, to deliver healthcare services remotely. This new modality is essential for rural and underserved populations where access to health care has previously been sacrificed due to geographic, infrastructural, and workforce limitations. Telehealth fills those gaps, allowing patients who live in remote areas to see their healthcare provider, obtain specialists' care, and receive timely intervention without making a long trip. It is essential to address the growing shortage of healthcare providers in rural environments, improve health outcomes *via* more consistent monitoring and early intervention, and lower patient and system-based costs. Moreover, telehealth serves as a medium for health education, disease prevention, and preparedness in times of crisis; thus, it is more accessible, equitable, and efficient for rural populations [4 - 6].

Current State of Healthcare in Rural Areas

Accessing medical care in rural areas continues to be a global problem, mainly due to geographic, socioeconomic, and systemic considerations. Rural populations have less access to medical facilities than their urban counterparts, with fewer hospitals, clinics, and diagnostic centres. The shortage of healthcare professionals, including general practitioners, specialists and nurses who often choose to work in urban areas due to better infrastructure, opportunities and quality of life, only contributes to the problem further [7].

Geographic isolation complicates things further since patients in rural areas often must travel great distances to reach even basic medical care. This is especially problematic when in need of emergency care, as delays in treatment can yield poor outcomes. Financial obstacles exacerbate these challenges, with rural populations typically having less income and less health insurance coverage, making many people unable to afford health care [8].

These chronic diseases, like diabetes, hypertension, and respiratory illnesses, result from a lack of preventive health care and low health education in these rural geographies due to limited infrastructural and financial resources. Moreover, advanced diagnostic tools, treatments, and specialists are in short supply.

Although efforts have been made to bridge these gaps through government programs and non-profit initiatives, the differences in healthcare access and quality between rural and urban populations remain a pressing concern. This highlights the imperative for innovative solutions, including telehealth, to address these challenges and enhance healthcare delivery for rural populations [9, 10].

Challenges Faced in Healthcare in Rural Areas

The challenges faced by rural healthcare are many and complex, making it difficult to provide equitable and efficient services in these areas. Accessibility is another critical challenge, considering that many rural areas are geographically isolated, which prevents residents from accessing primary or specialised medical care in a reasonable amount of time. Additionally, the number of healthcare centres is limited, and they are often poorly equipped for performing basic medical procedures and diagnostic tests. Poor connectivity, such as poor Internet and telecommunications infrastructure, also limits the adoption of modern solutions like telehealth. In rural areas, workforce shortages are critical barriers, with few doctors, nurses, and specialists willing to work there because resources are limited and the professional opportunities are less beneficial. Financial barriers, such as unaffordable care costs and widespread lack of health insurance, render healthcare unaffordable for many rural residents [11, 12]. Moreover, low health literacy and cultural beliefs tend to dissuade people from visiting healthcare facilities on time, which can result in an increased burden of existing chronic diseases and missed diagnoses. Disjointed health records, a digital divide around technology access, and uneven funding for rural health programs exacerbate these obstacles. Addressing these issues requires an integrated approach, including infrastructure growth, workforce preservation, affordable healthcare policies, and root innovation technologies [13 - 15]. Healthcare challenges faced in rural areas are summarised in Fig. (**1**).

BENEFITS OF TELEHEALTH

The benefits of telehealth help fill the gaps in traditional healthcare delivery and are incredibly impactful for rural and underserved communities. Its more significant benefits include better access to care, as telehealth can connect patients with healthcare providers, including specialists, from anywhere, removing the need to travel long distances. This geographical flexibility allows even those in rural locations access to timely and adequate care. It is also cost-effective, as patients can save on travel and time off work, and healthcare systems can achieve better resource allocation and lower overhead costs [16, 17].

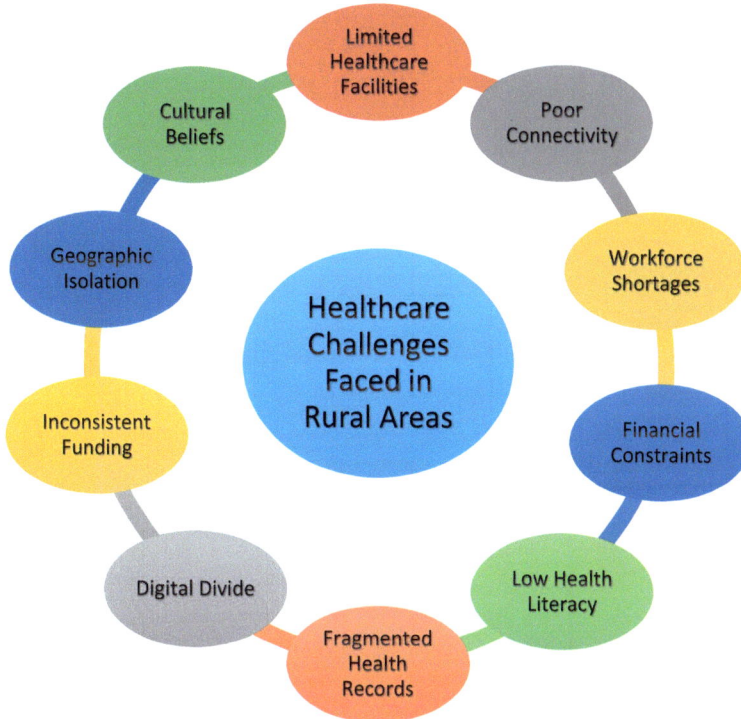

Fig. (1). Healthcare challenges faced in rural areas.

Telehealth also improves patient outcomes by allowing timely interventions and managing chronic diseases, such as diabetes and hypertension, through regular monitoring and follow-up. It introduced convenience and flexibility in consulting with providers from home and at a time that is around the patient's schedule, improving patient-centred care and access. Telehealth also supports health education and disease prevention, giving patients the information to make decisions, lead healthier lives, and prevent avoidable sicknesses [18].

Another advantage is continuity of care, which is ensured with telehealth platforms. These platforms often incorporate electronic health records (EHRs) to provide easy access to patient histories and facilitate better care coordination. Patients receive consistent follow-up care this way, leaving little gaps in treatment. Telehealth facilitates real-time consultations, prompt triage, and mental health support in emergencies or disasters when in-person visits are impossible [19].

Telehealth solutions can also help mitigate workforce issues by enabling urban healthcare providers to be dispersed to rural areas without the need to relocate. This allows local practitioners in underserved areas to work with specialists remotely, which, in turn, provides better care overall. Telehealth is revolutionising healthcare delivery into a more inclusive, efficient, and patient-centered system by closing gaps in accessibility, affordability, and quality [20].

APPLICATIONS OF TELEHEALTH IN RURAL COMMUNITIES

In rural communities where barriers to care due to limited physician supply, and poor infrastructure remain to improving health, telehealth has been a great new tool that can help improve healthcare delivery. Telemedicine has been used for a variety of applications in these communities, improving both access and quality of care [21, 22]. Applications of telehealth in rural communities are discussed below and summarised in Fig. (2).

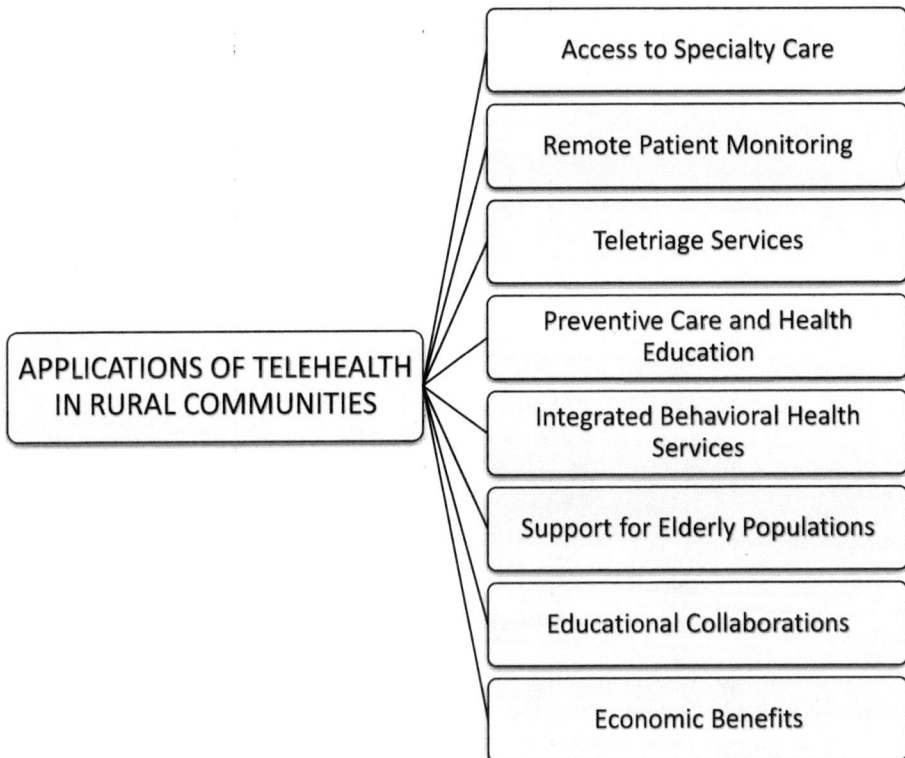

Fig. (2). Applications of telehealth in rural communities.

Access to Specialty Care

In many rural communities across the country, there are often significant barriers to getting specialty care because patients have to travel far from their homes to visit the urban centres where those specialists practice. Telehealth addresses this gap by allowing virtual consultations with specialists in numerous fields, including cardiology, endocrinology, and dermatology [23].

By enabling patients to access specialists from home, telehealth saves time and money on travel, which can be particularly difficult for those with chronic conditions or mobility difficulties. Research shows that patients who participate in telehealth consultations feel more satisfied and are more likely to comply with treatment recommendations.

Telehealth also fosters collaborative care models where primary care providers can work closely with specialists to manage complex cases. This integrated approach ensures that patients receive comprehensive care tailored to their needs [24].

Remote Patient Monitoring

Remotely monitored Patient (RMP) uses technology to transmit patient health data in real-time, allowing healthcare providers to oversee conditions such as hypertension, diabetes, or heart disease without requiring a visit to the clinic.

RPM devices monitor health markers, including blood pressure, glucometer readings, or heart rate, allowing the real-time transmission of this information to healthcare providers. When such abnormalities are detected, the leadless device continuously transmits data to allow for timely interventions and hopefully prevent decompensation that would require hospitalisation.

RPM empowers patients by letting them take charge of their health management. Many of them have very user-friendly interfaces, encouraging patients to know their metrics and actively participate in self-management efforts [25, 26].

Teletriage Services

Teletriage is a critical component of telehealth that assesses patient needs remotely before they seek care. This service helps prioritise healthcare resources efficiently.

In rural areas where emergency services may be limited or slow to respond, teletriage allows healthcare providers to evaluate the acuteness of a patient's condition *via* a phone call or video. This ensures that those requiring immediate attention receive it promptly, while others may be advised on home care options or scheduled for follow-up visits.

By directing patients to the appropriate level of care based on their needs, teletriage helps prevent overcrowding in emergency departments and clinics, ensuring that resources are utilised effectively [27, 28]. The workflow of the teletriage service is represented in Fig. (**3**).

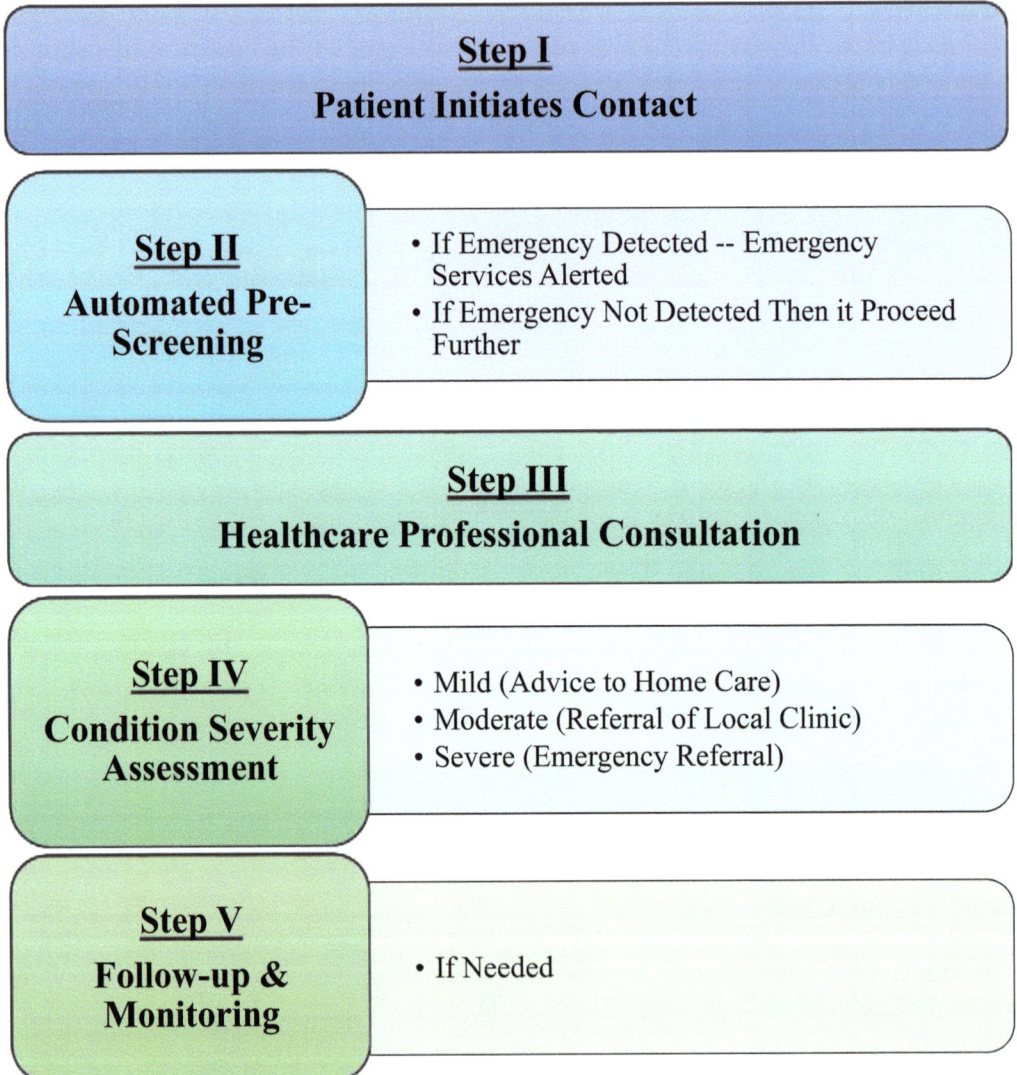

Step I
Patient Initiates Contact

Step II
Automated Pre-Screening
- If Emergency Detected -- Emergency Services Alerted
- If Emergency Not Detected Then it Proceed Further

Step III
Healthcare Professional Consultation

Step IV
Condition Severity Assessment
- Mild (Advice to Home Care)
- Moderate (Referral of Local Clinic)
- Severe (Emergency Referral)

Step V
Follow-up & Monitoring
- If Needed

Fig. (3). Flowchart of teletriage service working in a rural community.

Preventive Care and Health Education

Telehealth provides an essential tool for advancing prevention measures, focusing on addressing the prevalence of chronic conditions within rural areas. Thanks to telehealth platforms, healthcare providers can do health screenings for things like hypertension and diabetes without the patient having to come into their facility. Such screenings can help identify those at risk early enough, prior to the development of overt disease, and hopefully implement interventions that slow down or halt progression in terms of the natural history.

It provides an easy way for rural communities to implement health education programs for their unique requirements. Providers can offer webinars or virtual workshops on nutrition, physical activity, mental health awareness, and chronic disease management. This way, people are empowered with both the education and the means to be well [29, 30].

Integrated Behavioral Health Services

Accessing mental health services is particularly challenging in rural areas where stigma and provider shortages often deter individuals from seeking help. Mental health professionals offer therapy and psychiatric consultations remotely using telehealth. The availability of this service is essential in the treatment of depression, anxiety disorders, and substance abuse problems within rural settings.

Telehealth platforms, including community support programs, can route patients to peer support groups or counselling services. These programs create a support system and combat mental health crises with essential support [31, 32].

Support for Elderly Populations

The elderly living in rural areas face several mobility and accessibility obstacles with the availability of healthcare. Telehealth allows elderly patients with regular check-ups and chronic conditions to see their doctors without stepping out of the house. Some components of a virtual visit include medication management consults, fall risk assessments, and senior-specific rehab exercises.

In addition to medical consultations, telehealth platforms can function as social interaction hubs where seniors can participate in virtual group activities or attend support sessions. This reduces loneliness and isolation, which are very common among the elderly living in rural areas [33 - 35].

Educational Collaborations

Schools in rural areas increasingly recognise the value of telehealth in promoting student health and well-being. Working directly with healthcare providers, schools can provide students with telehealth services without even leaving campus. That includes routine health exams, mental health counselling and care for conditions like asthma or diabetes during the school day.

School-based telehealth provides immediate healthcare access and has health promotion implications for students' overall wellness. Well-educated students are more likely to be present in school regularly and do better academically [36, 37].

Economic Benefits

Telehealth has significant economic advantages for rural communities and the healthcare system. If patients can see healthcare providers virtually, it will save them travel costs and work time. Especially low-income families who can be deterred by the costs of transportation to receive care from entities that are in fewer places.

Rural healthcare facilities can also benefit from telehealth services as they expand their patient reach outside local populations. Increased patient volume can improve these facilities' financial sustainability while ensuring that residents receive necessary medical attention [38, 39].

OPTIMISED HEALTHCARE DELIVERY THROUGH TELEHEALTH

Telehealth has transformed the delivery of healthcare by improving efficiency, lowering costs, and expanding access to care, particularly in underserved communities [40]. Below is a comprehensive overview of the key aspects of telehealth that contribute to optimised healthcare delivery, also summarised in Fig. (4).

Cost-effectiveness and Efficiency

Telehealth has shown promise in saving costs across all kinds of healthcare settings. Studies have found that telehealth can help reduce healthcare spending by lessening the need for an office visit. It is often more costly because it involves higher transportation costs, which are only seen during facility hours and work lost to waiting in doctors' offices. The Veterans Health Administration reported that its remote patient monitoring program saved an average of $687 per patient per month instead of traditional care, primarily through decreased hospitalisations and emergency department visits. Moreover, some studies have indicated that the use of telemedicine was less expensive than usual care during outpatient consultation, and costs turned out to be considerably higher than traditional methods. Telehealth prevents health issues from escalating to the point where emergency care is needed for better outcomes and a lower overall cost [41, 42].

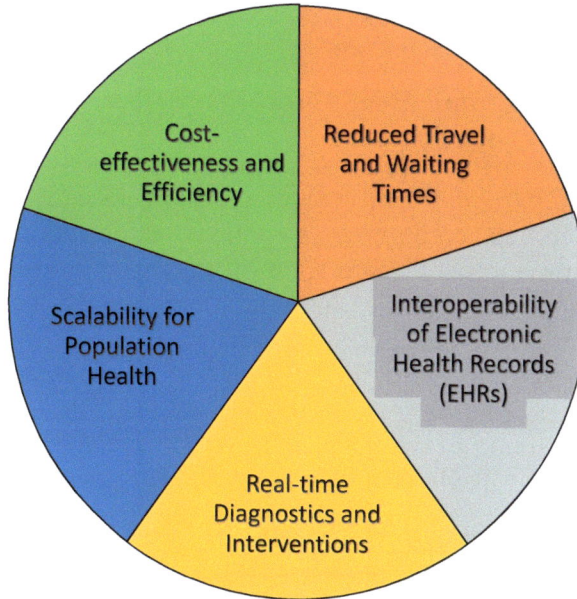

Fig. (4). Characteristics of telehealth that contribute to optimised healthcare delivery.

Reduced Travel and Waiting Times

One of the most significant advantages is that it addresses travel as a barrier for patients, which can be crucial in areas such as rural regions with very under-resourced healthcare facilities. Telehealth enables patients to be treated from home, reducing travel time and cost. It is of particular help to those who suffer from chronic diseases and have frequent follow-ups, but lack the mobility or means to travel back and forth. It also leads to shorter waiting times than traditional in-person consultations. This improves the experience for patients, who can get appointments sooner and without sitting on long waiting lists while allowing healthcare providers to make better use of their time [43, 44].

Scalability for Population Health

Telehealth provides a scalable option that is adjustable to the specific needs of any given population, representing an essential tool in the public health supply. Telehealth platforms reach a wide swath of the population regardless of geographic boundaries or controlled substances, giving people access to crucial care that they might not have otherwise gotten. This scalability is critical, especially during public health emergencies like the COVID-19 pandemic, where conventional healthcare delivery systems may get exhausted. Additionally, telehealth can provide targeted health programs and address population-specific health problems. For example, remote monitoring programs tailored to patients with chronic diseases such as diabetes or hypertension can provide for prevention and early intervention, limiting complications [45, 46].

Interoperability of Electronic Health Records (EHRs)

Integrating telehealth with Electronic Health Records (EHRs) enhances the continuity and coordination of care. Adopting interoperable EHR systems enables healthcare providers to communicate patient information across multiple platforms and inform a patient's care team of medical histories, treatment plans, and test results. This information dissemination quickly leads to data-driven decision-making and, therefore, more coordinated care. Real-time documentation using integrated EHRs will allow for better monitoring of patient outcomes and follow-up care conducted during telehealth encounters. These coordinated efforts help reduce the likelihood of mistakes and provide patients with a whole health package specific to their needs [47, 48].

Real-time Diagnostics and Interventions

Telehealth facilitates the timely detection of symptoms through highly advanced technologies like remote monitoring devices and mobile health apps. Wearable devices or home monitoring systems allow healthcare providers to track patients' vital signs and other health metrics in real time. This real-time data access enables early intervention when high blood pressure or erratic heart looping is detected, minimising the chances of something going wrong. Even better, telehealth platforms can allow for real-time feedback, increasing patient participation in their health management. This can include alerts based on monitored data (*e.g.*, reminding chronic patients about medication adherence or lifestyle changes). This engagement is intended to create a level of accountability that might translate into healthier choices [49, 50].

Real-time Diagnostics Data of Telehealth

Although telehealth can diagnose patients in real time and improve patient outcomes, it has dramatically improved healthcare delivery in rural areas. Rural patients who received remote patient monitoring had a 32% decrease in hospitalisations and a 14% decrease in ED visits, according to a study published in the Journal of Medical Internet Research. Additionally, studies showed that telemedicine consultations in rural India significantly reduce patient spending by 50%, costing only INR 1,000 (USD 13.5) per session as opposed to INR 2,000 (USD 27) for in-person visits [51].

Furthermore, a study of remote patient monitoring systems in rural Kentucky showed that 95% of non-emergency medical information was successfully sent with an average latency of roughly 13 hours when 30% of the population participated. These results highlight the real advantages of telehealth in improving access to healthcare and diagnostic services in rural areas [52].

CHALLENGES AND LIMITATIONS IN IMPLEMENTATION

Though telehealth has great potential to improve the healthcare provided to those in rural and other underserved communities, its implementation faces several challenges and limitations that must be addressed for maximum impact.

Technological Barriers

Reliability of the internet and gadgets is one of the key challenges in rural sectors. Infrastructure for high-speed internet is not widespread, and many patients may lack the required technology, such as cell phones or computers. Low digital literacy levels can further hinder the use of telehealth platforms, especially when patients do not have the skills necessary to navigate the technology [53, 54].

Regulatory and Reimbursement Issues

A telehealth solution is subject to different requirements depending on its region of operation. Many payers have reimbursement policies for telehealth services that are less robust than those for in-person visits. In areas short of funds, such as rural placements, this can create financial issues for the healthcare provider. Moreover, licensing restrictions could prevent healthcare providers from providing services within state or national boundaries and hence limit their power to consult specialists located in the local area [55, 56].

Limited Access to Healthcare Providers

Despite the potential of telehealth to link patients with specialists in other areas, many remote locations still lack nearby healthcare providers, including general practitioners. Even with telehealth, patients may experience delays in receiving care or face difficulties getting access to specialists willing to participate in remote consultations. This disparity in provider availability continues to challenge effective healthcare delivery, even with technological solutions [57, 58].

Socioeconomic and Cultural Barriers

Socioeconomic factors highly lead to the uptake of telehealth, mostly in rural and underserved communities. This can also worsen health inequities if low-income residents do not have the technology and internet needed for telehealth access.

Moreover, cultural limitations such as doubtfulness towards technology or unfamiliarity with telemedicine can lower its integration among populations, public education, and community outreach as a tool to overcome these barriers [59, 60].

Integration with Existing Healthcare Systems

Telehealth can be complicated when added to the healthcare infrastructure already in place. Rural healthcare facilities generally don't have the e-health Record (EHR) systems and IT infrastructure ready to provide telehealth services. Poor data integration between telehealth platforms and their existing EHRs can lead to broken care coordination, which limits the effectiveness of telehealth in rural areas [61, 62].

Emergency and Hands-on Care Limitations

Although telehealth is helpful in providing consultations and chronic care, it cannot be a complete solution for urgent care situations that may need immediate hands-on intervention like physical examinations or surgeries. Telehealth can not completely mimic the in-person immediate care provided by traditional clinical settings, and there will still be times when rural patients need to travel to urban centres for emergency or complex healthcare treatments.

Policymakers, health systems, and technology vendors need to collaborate to develop solutions that provide better access, improve the technological infrastructure, and ensure equitable and effective implementation of telehealth services in rural and underserved communities [63 - 65].

Infrastructure and Connectivity Issues

A significant obstacle to making telehealth programs work in rural areas is the shortage of solid internet and technological structures that will allow for efficient information exchange. This is essential for video consultations to be as smooth and high-quality as possible and for real-time data transmission. Patients cannot communicate effectively through telehealth, which means that many who choose or are forced into the new system cannot fully partake in telehealth services, widening the gap and reproducing further existing disparities. Moreover, some rural healthcare facilities have outdated or inadequate technology infrastructure that cannot be easily streamlined with telehealth solutions into their existing systems [66, 67].

Digital Literacy Among Rural Populations

However, Telehealth services require a base level of digital literacy, which can be a difficult hurdle to clear for the much older people in rural communities or anyone with little experience using technology. Some patients may struggle to use telehealth platforms, video calls or remote health monitoring equipment despite having internet access. This lack of digital readiness can often inhibit this population from taking full advantage of the available telehealth services, which decreases its effectiveness as a healthcare solution for rural populations [68].

Resistance to Adoption by Healthcare Providers

Telehealth is gaining popularity, but facilities in rural areas or operated by those who are set in their ways will not make the transition. The likely reasons behind such resistance are doubts about the success of remote consultations, a lack of awareness of telehealth technologies, or a belief that it is not fully equipped to offer care similar to an in-person visit. Additionally, healthcare providers in rural areas are already burdened with scarce resources, and implementing telehealth in their practice is just too much to add to that list [69, 70].

Legal and Regulatory Barriers

Telehealth must comply with complicated legal and regulatory landscapes, which can differ, even across states or internationally. Changes to telehealth reimbursement policies over the past year have presented challenges to many rural healthcare providers, who often either cannot cover the full costs of providing more consultations without localising care or face limits on what services are deemed eligible for reimbursement. Licensing issues frequently prohibit healthcare providers from offering telehealth services to patients in other states or regions. Telehealth regulations also differ from state to state, making it difficult for a healthcare provider to provide care across the border and restricting access to additional specialists and services.

These challenges pose the need for targeted efforts to ensure infrastructure development, promotion and acceptance by healthcare providers, digital literacy within the ecosystem, and legal and security issues. Telehealth, working together with its partners, will be a game-changing vehicle for providing quality healthcare to rural and underserved communities [71, 72].

CASE STUDIES AND SUCCESS STORIES

Global Examples of Telehealth Adoption in Rural Areas

Several countries worldwide have successfully adopted telehealth to address the healthcare needs of rural populations, serving as models for other regions.

Australia's National Telehealth Strategy

Through Australia's broad telehealth program, these services are being provided to rural and remote areas. There is a government-funded "Telehealth Medicare Benefits Schedule" (MBS) that allows patients in rural areas to have consultations with GPs and other specialists *via* video. The benefits include reducing the burden on travel and thus making for easy special care availability, leading to improved results for chronic disease and mental health patients and frequent consults [73, 74].

Canada's Virtual Care in Northern Communities

Canada has also advanced in the sense of virtual healthcare for its northern remote regions. Video conferencing also brings some benefits, like the region of Northern Health Authority, which has the means to connect patients with specialist health care through programs such as telehealth services. The services have made care more accessible and timely, especially for Indigenous populations and those residing in remote locales. For instance, Canadians depend on telehealth services to receive mental health support, chronic disease management, and primary preventive care [75, 76].

India's eSanjeevani Telemedicine Platform

In India, the eSanjeevani platform is one of a kind that provides telemedicine services to the rural and underserved population. An initiative of the Ministry of Health and Family Welfare, the service connects remote patients with doctors for a virtual consultation. It has been considerably impacted by delivering primary healthcare to villages, addressing general health-related issues of patients who use the system, maternal care, and chronic disease management [77, 78].

National Programs Focused on Rural Telemedicine

National programs dedicated to telemedicine have been instrumental in expanding access to healthcare in rural areas, with many providing comprehensive solutions for healthcare delivery.

United States: The Rural Health Care Program (Rural Healthcare Funding Program)

The Rural Health Care Program of the Federal Communications Commission (FCC) allows for subsidies paid to rural health care providers for using telemedicine/telehealth services within the U.S. The program has allowed towns access to superfast broadband for rural clinics and hospitals while receiving remote diagnostics equipment and telehealth platforms. This has been very important in fields like behavioural health, where there are not a lot of mental health professionals in all the places that need them. The initiative has resulted in better outcomes for patients with mental illness, chronic conditions, and urgent care requirements [79, 80].

United Kingdom: NHS Virtual Consultation Services

The UK's National Health Service (NHS) introduced virtual appointment systems to address disparities between urban and rural areas. In some remote regions, patients can get information, book consultations, and even care without having to travel across the country by digital health initiatives such as NHS 111. The pandemic has sped up the adoption of telehealth areas of the NHS. This model is being used as a mainstream approach to healthcare delivery, especially in rural and underserved regions [81, 82].

Success Metrics and Lessons Learned

Several factors, including access to care, patient satisfaction, cost savings, and health outcomes, typically measure the success of telehealth programs in rural areas.

Access to Care

Telehealth has made a massive difference in rural communities, allowing residents to immediately skip the long drive and speak with a medical provider. For example, in Australia, telehealth services have enabled patients in remote areas to consult with specialists who would otherwise be inaccessible [83, 84].

Patient Satisfaction

Research and surveys conducted around the globe suggest that rural patients express high satisfaction levels in receiving their care *via* telehealth. In northern communities in Canada, patients are more satisfied with telehealth for its convenience and the fact that they can do it from home. Mental health services had the highest proportion of satisfied patients, which could be because going for an in-person visit can carry a certain stigma, coupled with privacy concerns [85].

Cost Savings

Studies have indicated that telehealth programs reduce the overall costs of healthcare delivery. In the US, rural telehealth services that reduced travel to see a doctor resulted in fewer in-person visits, which cost both patients and providers. This has shown promising results in chronic disease management and preventative care, decreasing hospital readmissions and ER visits [86].

Health Outcomes

Telehealth has been shown to have beneficial health impacts; examples can even be found internationally in countries like the UK and India. In India, telehealth has increased immunisation and reduced maternal and infant mortality in rural areas. In rural areas, treating chronic diseases *via* telehealth can increase consumer adherence to treatment plans, lower the likelihood of complications, and improve long-term health outcomes [87].

Lessons Learned

Technology Infrastructure

Success is heavily dependent on the availability of reliable internet and technology infrastructure. Telehealth cannot be adopted without efficient and affordable technology for healthcare providers and patients [88].

Training and Support

Telehealth platforms require proper training for patients and healthcare providers alike. Digital literacy programs for patients and technical training for healthcare providers funded through investment in telehealth systems have been used to increase confidence and effectiveness of telehealth use, demonstrating substantial benefit in some states [89].

Policy and Regulatory Support

It is also necessary to provide government policies specific to telehealth reimbursement and regulations allowing the safe and effective operation of remote care. Successful programs require deep partnerships with public health agencies, technology providers, and healthcare professionals to navigate regulatory challenges for both patient needs and continuity of care [90].

FUTURE DIRECTIONS

The future of telehealth in underserved populations, as it continues to advance, will be defined by applying various emerging technologies, advancing policies, and creating a sustainable foundation so that adoption can reach its maximum potential. Using blockchain technology to store health data can provide an efficient, secure, and private system for patients to manage their records. Not only will it solve the issue of data breaches, but it will also help to gain confidence among rural people. However, IoT helps in healthcare monitoring and allows health data collection remotely through those connected devices to enhance chronic disease management and enable timely interventions without patients needing to visit physically [91].

From a policy perspective, governments and stakeholders will need to develop regulations and frameworks that facilitate the adoption of telehealth but ensure its quality and safety. Recommendations for policy should include expanding access to broadband infrastructure in rural areas, providing incentives for telehealth adoption by providers, and removing of barriers to wide-spread reimbursement of telehealth as a reimbursable component of care. Additionally, it is crucial to establish clear guidelines for using telehealth across state or national borders, enabling wider access to specialists [92].

Incentives have also been recommended as a tool to increase healthcare provider participation. These incentives may include financial reimbursements, training programs, and technical support. Ensuring healthcare professionals in underserved areas have access to ongoing education on telehealth platforms and are compensated fairly for remote consultations will help increase provider engagement [93].

Telehealth strategies should ultimately prioritise sustainability and long-term planning throughout the implementation process. This includes integrating telehealth services into the overall healthcare system, sustaining technological infrastructure, and collaboration between government sectors with private companies, and healthcare systems. Promoting public-private partnerships can help fund and scale telehealth services, while continuous assessment and feedback from rural communities will be essential to refine and improve telehealth services over time. By focusing on these future directions, telehealth can become a transformative tool for improving healthcare accessibility and equity in underserved communities [94, 95].

CONCLUSION

Telehealth can address these gaps and enable effective healthcare delivery to rural and underserved communities by offering more accessible care solutions that are convenient for the patient and sustainable in the long term. Telehealth supports healthcare providers in reaching and intervening sooner among populations facing barriers due to geographic isolation, access restrictions or the prohibitive nature of healthcare costs, enabling patients to understand and manage chronic diseases more effectively. Telehealth can increase rural healthcare's efficiency, access, and patient-centeredness by using virtual consultations, remote monitoring, and health education. Nevertheless, while the advantages are sizable, a few obstacles have to be overcome if telehealth is to be effectively deployed in these contexts. The nature of those hurdles will vary significantly and include filling infrastructure gaps, increasing digital literacy, managing regulatory obstacles, and addressing provider resistance to new ways of care delivery. In addition, incorporating innovative technologies like Blockchain and the Internet of Things (IoT) will enhance telehealth security and make them more efficient now and in the future for whole-person care. Telehealth will continue to play a central role in bridging healthcare disparities, provided that policies, incentives, and sustainable strategies are implemented. Collaboration across governments, healthcare entities, and technology development is critical to mobilising the continued expansion of telehealth services, with particular attention drawn to rural and underserved populations. By doing so, telehealth can vastly improve healthcare equity, streamline care delivery, and drive meaningful improvements in health outcomes for the millions of people within these communities.

CONSENT FOR PUBLICATON

All authors have given their consent for publication. The authors authorised Mohammad Mansoor to handle all correspondence.

ACKNOWLEDGEMENTS

Authors are highly thankful to their Universities/Colleges for providing library facilities for the literature survey.

REFERENCES

[1]   Lokken TG, Blegen RN, Hoff MD, Demaerschalk BM. Overview for implementing telemedicine services in a large integrated multispecialty health care system. Telemed J E Health 2020; 26(4): 382-7.
        [http://dx.doi.org/10.1089/tmj.2019.0079] [PMID: 31433261]

[2]   McGee R, Tangalos EG. Delivery of health care to the underserved: potential contributions of telecommunications technology. Consensus conference entitled telemedicine and access to care. Mayo Clin Proc 1994; 69(12): 1131-36.

[http://dx.doi.org/10.1016/S0025-6196(12)65763-2]

[3]   Schutte-Rodin S. Telehealth, telemedicine, and obstructive sleep apnea. Sleep Med Clin 2020; 15(3): 359-75.
        [http://dx.doi.org/10.1016/j.jsmc.2020.05.003] [PMID: 32762969]

[4]   Haleem A, Javaid M, Singh RP, Suman R. Telemedicine for healthcare: Capabilities, features, barriers, and applications. Sens Int 2021; 2: 100117.

[5]   Anawade PA, Sharma D, Gahane S. A Comprehensive Review on Exploring the Impact of Telemedicine on Healthcare Accessibility. Cureus 2024; 16(3): e55996.
        [http://dx.doi.org/10.7759/cureus.55996] [PMID: 38618307]

[6]   Chen J, Amaize A, Barath D. Evaluating telehealth adoption and related barriers among hospitals in rural and urban areas. J Rural Health 2021; 37(4): 801-11.
        [http://dx.doi.org/10.1111/jrh.12534] [PMID: 33180363]

[7]   Weinhold I, Gurtner S. Understanding shortages of sufficient health care in rural areas. Health Policy 2014; 118(2): 201-14.
        [http://dx.doi.org/10.1016/j.healthpol.2014.07.018] [PMID: 25176511]

[8]   Moscovice I, Rosenblatt R. Quality-of-care challenges for rural health. J Rural Health 2000; 16(2): 168-76.
        [http://dx.doi.org/10.1111/j.1748-0361.2000.tb00451.x] [PMID: 10981369]

[9]   Patil AV, Somasundaram KV, Goyal RC. Current health scenario in rural India. Aust J Rural Health 2002; 10(2): 129-35.
        [http://dx.doi.org/10.1111/j.1440-1584.2002.tb00022.x] [PMID: 12047509]

[10]   Ricketts TC. The changing nature of rural health care. Annu Rev Public Health 2000; 21(1): 639-57.
        [http://dx.doi.org/10.1146/annurev.publhealth.21.1.639] [PMID: 10884968]

[11]   Ford DM. Four persistent rural healthcare challenges. Healthc Manage Forum 2016; 29(6): 243–46.
        [http://dx.doi.org/10.1177/0840470416658903]

[12]   Panagariya DA. The challenges and innovative solutions to rural health dilemmas. Ann Neurosci 2014; 21(4): 125-7.
        [http://dx.doi.org/10.5214/ans.0972.7531.210401] [PMID: 25452670]

[13]   Nelson WA. The challenges of rural health care. In: Klugman CM, Dalinis PM, Eds. Ethical issues in rural health care. Baltimore (MD): Johns Hopkins University Press 2008; pp. 34–59.

[14]   Coughlin SS, Clary C, Johnson JA, *et al.* Continuing challenges in rural health in the United States. J Environ Health Sci 2019; 5(2): 90-2.
        [PMID: 32104722]

[15]   Bailey JM. The top 10 rural issues for health care reform. Center for Rural Affairs 2009; 2(1): 1-8.

[16]   Gajarawala SN, Pelkowski JN. Telehealth benefits and barriers. J Nurse Pract 2021; 17(2): 218-21.
        [http://dx.doi.org/10.1016/j.nurpra.2020.09.013] [PMID: 33106751]

[17]   Moffatt JJ, Eley DS. The reported benefits of telehealth for rural Australians. Aust Health Rev 2010; 34(3): 276-81.
        [http://dx.doi.org/10.1071/AH09794] [PMID: 20797357]

[18]   Snoswell CL, Smith AC, Page M, Scuffham P, Caffery LJ. Quantifying the societal benefits from telehealth: productivity and reduced travel. Value Health Reg Issues 2022; 28: 61-6.
        [http://dx.doi.org/10.1016/j.vhri.2021.07.007] [PMID: 34800833]

[19]   Lillicrap L, Hunter C, Goldswain P. Improving geriatric care and reducing hospitalisations in regional and remote areas: The benefits of telehealth. J Telemed Telecare 2021; 27(7): 397-408.
        [http://dx.doi.org/10.1177/1357633X19881588] [PMID: 31645171]

[20]   Mahtta D, Daher M, Lee MT, Sayani S, Shishehbor M, Virani SS. Promise and perils of telehealth in

the current era. Curr Cardiol Rep 2021; 23(9): 115.
[http://dx.doi.org/10.1007/s11886-021-01544-w] [PMID: 34269884]

[21]   Butzner M, Cuffee Y. Telehealth interventions and outcomes across rural communities in the United States: narrative review. J Med Internet Res 2021; 23(8): e29575.
[http://dx.doi.org/10.2196/29575] [PMID: 34435965]

[22]   Marcin JP, Shaikh U, Steinhorn RH. Addressing health disparities in rural communities using telehealth. Pediatr Res 2016; 79(1-2): 169-76.
[http://dx.doi.org/10.1038/pr.2015.192] [PMID: 26466080]

[23]   Uddin J, Fariha T, Shumi SS. Bridging the gap: expanding telehealth services to address rural health disparities. Int J Sci Res Multidiscip Stud 2024; 10(7): 50–7.

[24]   Bagchi AD. Expansion of telehealth across the rural-urban continuum. State Local Gov Rev 2019; 51(4): 250-8.
[http://dx.doi.org/10.1177/0160323X20929053]

[25]   Serrano LP, Maita KC, Avila FR, *et al.* Benefits and challenges of remote patient monitoring as perceived by health care practitioners: a systematic review. Perm J 2023; 27(4): 100-11.
[http://dx.doi.org/10.7812/TPP/23.022] [PMID: 37735970]

[26]   Ferdausi NS, Fatema NK, Mahmud NM, Hoque NR, Ali NM. Transforming telehealth with Artificial Intelligence: Predictive and diagnostic advances in remote patient care. World J Adv Eng Technol Sci 2025; 16(1): 355-65.
[http://dx.doi.org/10.30574/wjaets.2025.16.1.1216]

[27]   Haimi M, Wheeler SQ. Safety in teletriage by nurses and physicians in the United States and Israel: narrative review and qualitative study JMIR Human Factors 2024; 11(1): e50676.
[http://dx.doi.org/10.2196/50676] [PMID: 38526526]

[28]   Farzandipour M, Nabovati E, Sharif R. The effectiveness of tele-triage during the COVID-19 pandemic: A systematic review and narrative synthesis. J Telemed Telecare 2024; 30(9): 1367-75.
[http://dx.doi.org/10.1177/1357633X221150278] [PMID: 36683438]

[29]   Maroju RG, Choudhari SG, Shaikh MK, Borkar SK, Mendhe H. Role of telemedicine and digital technology in public health in India: a narrative review. Cureus 2023; 15(3): e35986.
[http://dx.doi.org/10.7759/cureus.35986] [PMID: 37050980]

[30]   Stoltzfus M, Kaur A, Chawla A, Gupta V, Anamika FNU, Jain R. The role of telemedicine in healthcare: an overview and update. Egypt J Intern Med 2023; 35(1): 49.
[http://dx.doi.org/10.1186/s43162-023-00234-z]

[31]   Nelson D, Inghels M, Kenny A, *et al.* Mental health professionals and telehealth in a rural setting: a cross sectional survey. BMC Health Serv Res 2023; 23(1): 200.
[http://dx.doi.org/10.1186/s12913-023-09083-6] [PMID: 36849933]

[32]   Connolly SL, Miller CJ, Gifford AL, Charness ME. Perceptions and use of telehealth among mental health, primary, and speciality care clinicians during the COVID-19 pandemic. JAMA Netw Open 2022; 5(6): e2216401.
[http://dx.doi.org/10.1001/jamanetworkopen.2022.16401] [PMID: 35671053]

[33]   Hunter I, Lockhart C, Rao V, Tootell B, Wong S. Enabling rural telehealth for older adults in underserved rural communities: focus group study. JMIR Form Res 2022; 6(11): e35864.
[http://dx.doi.org/10.2196/35864] [PMID: 36331533]

[34]   Fox K. Barriers to elderly accessibility to healthcare in rural areas. Bachelor's thesis. Murray (KY): Murray State University 2024.

[35]   Dykgraaf SH, Desborough J, Sturgiss E, Parkinson A, Dut GM, Kidd M. Older people, the digital divide and use of telehealth during the COVID-19 pandemic. Aust J Gen Pract 2022; 51(9): 721-4.
[http://dx.doi.org/10.31128/AJGP-03-22-6358] [PMID: 36045630]

[36] Young TL, Ireson C. Effectiveness of school-based telehealth care in urban and rural elementary schools. Pediatrics 2003; 112(5): 1088-94.
[http://dx.doi.org/10.1542/peds.112.5.1088] [PMID: 14595051]

[37] Rettinger L, Putz P, Aichinger L, *et al.* Telehealth education in allied health care and nursing: Web-based cross-sectional survey of students' perceived knowledge, skills, attitudes, and experience. JMIR Med Educ 2024; 10(1): e51112.
[http://dx.doi.org/10.2196/51112] [PMID: 38512310]

[38] Snoswell CL, North JB, Caffery LJ. Economic advantages of telehealth and virtual health practitioners: return on investment analysis. JMIR Perioperative Medicine 2020; 3(1): e15688.
[http://dx.doi.org/10.2196/15688] [PMID: 33393922]

[39] Rajkumar E, Gopi A, Joshi A, *et al.* Applications, benefits and challenges of telehealth in India during COVID-19 pandemic and beyond: a systematic review. BMC Health Serv Res 2023; 23(1): 7.
[http://dx.doi.org/10.1186/s12913-022-08970-8] [PMID: 36597088]

[40] Knudsen KE, Willman C, Winn R. Optimizing the use of telemedicine in oncology care: postpandemic opportunities. Clin Cancer Res 2021; 27(4): 933-6.
[http://dx.doi.org/10.1158/1078-0432.CCR-20-3758] [PMID: 33229457]

[41] Snoswell CL, Taylor ML, Comans TA, Smith AC, Gray LC, Caffery LJ. Determining if telehealth can reduce health system costs is a scoping review. J Med Internet Res 2020; 22(10): e17298.
[http://dx.doi.org/10.2196/17298] [PMID: 33074157]

[42] Lee JS, Bhatt A, Pollack LM, et al. Telehealth use during the early COVID-19 public health emergency and subsequent health care costs and utilization. Health Aff Sch 2024; 2(1): qxae001.

[43] Francke JA, Groden P, Ferrer C, *et al.* Remote enrollment into a telehealth-delivering patient portal: Barriers faced in an urban population during the COVID-19 pandemic. Health Technol (Berl) 2022; 12(1): 227-38.
[http://dx.doi.org/10.1007/s12553-021-00614-x] [PMID: 34777935]

[44] Cooper S. Opinion leaders' perspective of the benefits and barriers in telemedicine: a grounded theory study of telehealth in the Midwest. Q Rev Distance Educ 2015; 16(1): 25.

[45] Milat A, Newson R, King L, *et al.* A guide to scaling up population health interventions. Public Health Res Pract 2016; 26(1): e2611604.
[http://dx.doi.org/10.17061/phrp2611604] [PMID: 26863167]

[46] Ben Charif A, Zomahoun HTV, Gogovor A, *et al.* Tools for assessing the scalability of innovations in health: a systematic review. Health Res Policy Syst 2022; 20(1): 34.
[http://dx.doi.org/10.1186/s12961-022-00830-5] [PMID: 35331260]

[47] Bahga A, Madisetti VK. A cloud-based approach for interoperable electronic health records (EHRs). IEEE J Biomed Health Inform 2013; 17(5): 894-906.
[http://dx.doi.org/10.1109/JBHI.2013.2257818] [PMID: 25055368]

[48] Jardim SVB. The electronic health record and its contribution to healthcare information systems interoperability. Procedia Technol 2013; 9: 940-8.
[http://dx.doi.org/10.1016/j.protcy.2013.12.105]

[49] Udegbe FC, Nwankwo EI, Igwama GT, Olaboye JA. Real-time data integration in diagnostic devices for predictive modelling of infectious disease outbreaks. Comput Sci IT Res J 2023; 4(3): 525–45.

[50] Messacar K, Hurst AL, Child J, *et al.* Clinical impact and provider acceptability of real-time antimicrobial stewardship decision support for rapid diagnostics in children with positive blood culture results. J Pediatric Infect Dis Soc 2017; 6(3): 267-74.
[PMID: 27543412]

[51] Chandrakar M. Telehealth and digital tools enhancing healthcare access in rural systems. Discover Public Health 2024; 21(1): 144.

[http://dx.doi.org/10.1186/s12982-024-00271-1]

[52] Max-Onakpoya E, Adebayo O, Ojo M, Oluwaranti A, Adedokun E. Augmenting cloud connectivity with opportunistic networks for rural remote patient monitoring. In: 2020 International Conference on Computing, Networking and Communications (ICNC); 2020; Big Island (HI): IEEE. pp. 920–6.
[http://dx.doi.org/10.1109/ICNC47757.2020.9049733]

[53] Ezeamii VC, Okobi OE, Wambai-Sani H, *et al.* Revolutionizing healthcare: How telemedicine is improving patient outcomes and expanding access to care. Cureus 2024; 16(7): e63881.
[http://dx.doi.org/10.7759/cureus.63881] [PMID: 39099901]

[54] Graves JM, Abshire DA, Amiri S, Mackelprang JL. Disparities in technology and broadband internet access across rurality: implications for health and education. Fam Community Health 2021; 44(4): 257-65.
[http://dx.doi.org/10.1097/FCH.0000000000000306] [PMID: 34269696]

[55] Day SC, Day G, Keller M, *et al.* Personalized implementation of video telehealth for rural veterans (PIVOT-R). mHealth 2021; 7: 24.
[http://dx.doi.org/10.21037/mhealth.2020.03.02] [PMID: 33898593]

[56] Kruse CS, Williams K, Bohls J, Shamsi W. Telemedicine and health policy: A systematic review. Health Policy Technol 2021; 10(1): 209-29.
[http://dx.doi.org/10.1016/j.hlpt.2020.10.006]

[57] Mathew S, Fitts MS, Liddle Z, *et al.* Telehealth in remote Australia: a supplementary tool or an alternative model of care replacing face-to-face consultations? BMC Health Serv Res 2023; 23(1): 341.
[http://dx.doi.org/10.1186/s12913-023-09265-2] [PMID: 37020234]

[58] Amjad A, Kordel P, Fernandes G. A review on innovation in the healthcare sector (telehealth) through artificial intelligence. Sustainability (Basel) 2023; 15(8): 6655.
[http://dx.doi.org/10.3390/su15086655]

[59] Cuadros DF, Moreno CM, Miller FD, Omori R, MacKinnon NJ. Assessing Access to Digital Services in Health Care–Underserved Communities in the United States: A Cross-Sectional Study. Mayo Clinic Proceedings: Digital Health 2023; 1(3): 217-25.
[http://dx.doi.org/10.1016/j.mcpdig.2023.04.004] [PMID: 40206610]

[60] Haimi M. The tragic paradoxical effect of telemedicine on healthcare disparities- a time for redemption: a narrative review. BMC Med Inform Decis Mak 2023; 23(1): 95.
[http://dx.doi.org/10.1186/s12911-023-02194-4] [PMID: 37193960]

[61] Zhang X, Saltman R. Impact of electronic health record interoperability on telehealth service outcomes. JMIR Med Inform 2022; 10(1): e31837.
[http://dx.doi.org/10.2196/31837] [PMID: 34890347]

[62] Banbury A, Smith AC, Mehrotra A, Page M, Caffery LJ. A comparison study between metropolitan and rural hospital-based telehealth activity to inform adoption and expansion. J Telemedicine and Telecare. 2023; 29(7): 540-51.

[63] Rowther AA, Mehmood A, Razzak JA, Atiq H, Castillo-Salgado C, Saleem HT. "You can only help them save the patient once they trust you": Clinician perspectives and theories of use of a pediatric emergency teleconsultation program. SSM - Qualitative Research in Health 2022; 2: 100150.
[http://dx.doi.org/10.1016/j.ssmqr.2022.100150]

[64] Ärlebrant L, Dubois H, Creutzfeldt J, Edin-Liljegren A. Emergency care *via* video consultation: interviews on patient experiences from rural community hospitals in northern Sweden. Int J Emerg Med 2024; 17(1): 109.
[http://dx.doi.org/10.1186/s12245-024-00703-4] [PMID: 39227787]

[65] Warner I. Introduction to telehealth home care. Home Healthc Nurse 1996; 14(10): 791-2.
[http://dx.doi.org/10.1097/00004045-199610000-00006] [PMID: 9052063]

[66] Arora S, Huda RK, Verma S, Khetan M, Sangwan RK. Challenges, barriers, and facilitators in telemedicine implementation in India: a scoping review. Cureus 2024; 16(8): e67388.
[http://dx.doi.org/10.7759/cureus.67388] [PMID: 39310647]

[67] Gurupur VP, Miao Z. A brief analysis of challenges in implementing telehealth in a rural setting. mHealth 2022; 8: 17.
[http://dx.doi.org/10.21037/mhealth-21-38] [PMID: 35449506]

[68] Rasekaba TM, Pereira P, Rani G V, Johnson R, McKechnie R, Blackberry I. Exploring telehealth readiness in a resource-limited setting: digital and health literacy among older people in Rural India (DAHLIA). Geriatrics (Basel) 2022; 7(2): 28.
[http://dx.doi.org/10.3390/geriatrics7020028] [PMID: 35314600]

[69] Gagnon MP, Ngangue P, Payne-Gagnon J, Desmartis M. m-Health adoption by healthcare professionals: a systematic review. J Am Med Inform Assoc 2016; 23(1): 212-20.
[http://dx.doi.org/10.1093/jamia/ocv052] [PMID: 26078410]

[70] Hale TM, Kvedar JC. Privacy and security concerns in telehealth. Virtual Mentor 2014; 16(12): 981-5.
[PMID: 25493367]

[71] Rowthorn V, Plum AJ, Zervos J. Legal and regulatory barriers to reverse innovation. Ann Glob Health 2017; 82(6): 991-1000.
[http://dx.doi.org/10.1016/j.aogh.2016.10.013] [PMID: 28314501]

[72] Lahey W, Currie R. Regulatory and medico-legal barriers to interprofessional practice. J Interprof Care 2005; 19(sup1): 197-223.
[http://dx.doi.org/10.1080/13561820500083188]

[73] Gill M. A national telehealth strategy for Australia–for discussion. Australian National Consultative Committee on Electronic Health. 2011 Nov.

[74] Taylor A, Caffery LJ, Gesesew HA, *et al.* How Australian health care services adapted to telehealth during the COVID-19 pandemic: a survey of telehealth professionals. Front Public Health 2021; 9: 648009.
[http://dx.doi.org/10.3389/fpubh.2021.648009] [PMID: 33718325]

[75] Buyting R, Melville S, Chatur H, *et al.* Virtual care with digital technologies for rural Canadians living with cardiovascular disease. CJC open. 2022 Feb 1;4(2):133-47.
[http://dx.doi.org/10.1016/j.cjco.2021.09.027]

[76] Gillespie J. Health disparities for Canada's remote and northern residents: Can COVID-19 help level the field? J Bioeth Inq 2023; 20(2): 207-13.
[http://dx.doi.org/10.1007/s11673-023-10245-8] [PMID: 37093411]

[77] Manjunatha N, Suhas S, Kumar CN, Math SB. E-sanjeevani: A pathbreaking telemedicine initiativefrom India. J Psychiatry Spectrum 2022; 1(2): 111-6.
[http://dx.doi.org/10.4103/jopsys.jopsys_8_21]

[78] Dastidar BG, Jani AR, Suri S, Nagaraja VH. Reimagining India's national telemedicine service to improve access to care. Lancet Reg Health Southeast Asia 2025; 30: 100480.
[http://dx.doi.org/10.1016/j.lansea.2024.100480]

[79] Beatty K, Heffernan M, Hale N, Meit M. Funding and service delivery in rural and urban local US health departments in 2010 and 2016. Am J Public Health 2020; 110(9): 1293-9.
[http://dx.doi.org/10.2105/AJPH.2020.305757] [PMID: 32673110]

[80] DeLeon PH, Wakefield M, Schultz AJ, Williams J, VandenBos GR. Rural America: Unique opportunities for health care delivery and health services research. Am Psychol 1989; 44(10): 1298-306.
[http://dx.doi.org/10.1037/0003-066X.44.10.1298] [PMID: 2802362]

[81] Quinn LM, Davies MJ, Hadjiconstantinou M. Virtual consultations and the role of technology during

the COVID-19 pandemic for people with type 2 diabetes: the UK perspective. J Med Internet Res 2020; 22(8): e21609.
[http://dx.doi.org/10.2196/21609] [PMID: 32716898]

[82]   O'Cathail M, Sivanandan MA, Diver C, Patel P, Christian J. The use of patient-facing teleconsultations in the national health service: a scoping review. JMIR Med Inform 2020; 8(3): e15380.
[http://dx.doi.org/10.2196/15380] [PMID: 32175911]

[83]   Seibert DC, Guthrie JT, Adamo G. Improving learning outcomes: integration of standardized patients & telemedicine technology. Nurs Educ Perspect 2004; 25(5): 232-7.
[PMID: 15508562]

[84]   Sreelatha O, S Ve R. Teleophthalmology: improving patient outcomes? Clin Ophthalmol 2016; 10: 285-95.
[http://dx.doi.org/10.2147/OPTH.S80487] [PMID: 26929592]

[85]   Harkey LC, Jung SM, Newton ER, Patterson A. Patient satisfaction with telehealth in rural settings: a systematic review. Int J Telerehabil 2020; 12(2): 53-64.
[http://dx.doi.org/10.5195/ijt.2020.6303] [PMID: 33520095]

[86]   Jungbauer WN Jr, Gudipudi R, Brennan E, Melvin CL, Pecha PP. The cost impact of telehealth interventions in pediatric surgical specialities: a systematic review. J Pediatr Surg 2023; 58(8): 1527-33.
[http://dx.doi.org/10.1016/j.jpedsurg.2022.10.008] [PMID: 36379748]

[87]   Parthasarathi A, George T, Kalimuth MB, *et al.* Exploring the potential of telemedicine for improved primary healthcare in India: a comprehensive review. Lancet Reg Health Southeast Asia 2024; 27: 100431.
[http://dx.doi.org/10.1016/j.lansea.2024.100431]

[88]   Sharma A, Pruthi M, Sageena G. Adoption of telehealth technologies: an approach to improving healthcare system. Transl Med Commun 2022; 7(1): 20.
[http://dx.doi.org/10.1186/s41231-022-00125-5] [PMID: 35967767]

[89]   Fitzpatrick PJ. Improving health literacy using the power of digital communications to achieve better health outcomes for patients and practitioners. Front in Digi Heal 2023; 5: 1264780.
[http://dx.doi.org/10.3389/fdgth.2023.1264780] [PMID: 38046643]

[90]   Nicol Turner Lee JK, Roberts J. Removing regulatory barriers to telehealth before and after COVID-19. Brookings Institution. 2020 May 6.

[91]   Damaševičius R, Abayomi-Alli OO. The future of telemedicine: emerging technologies, challenges, and opportunities. In: Gaur L, Jhanjhi NZ, Eds. Metaverse Applications for Intelligent Healthcare. Hershey (PA): IGI Global 2023; pp. 306–338.

[92]   Stoumpos AI, Kitsios F, Talias MA. Digital transformation in healthcare: technology acceptance and its applications. Int J Environ Res Public Health 2023; 20(4): 3407.
[http://dx.doi.org/10.3390/ijerph20043407] [PMID: 36834105]

[93]   Adeghe EP, Okolo CA, Ojeyinka OT. A review of emerging trends in telemedicine: Healthcare delivery transformations. Int J Life Sci Res Arch 2024; 6(1): 137-47.
[http://dx.doi.org/10.53771/ijlsra.2024.6.1.0040]

[94]   Yeroushalmi S, Maloni H, Costello K, Wallin MT. Telemedicine and multiple sclerosis: A comprehensive literature review. J Telemed Telecare 2020; 26(7-8): 400-13.
[http://dx.doi.org/10.1177/1357633X19840097] [PMID: 31042118]

[95]   Ryu S. History of telemedicine: evolution, context, and transformation. Healthc Inform Res 2010; 16(1): 65-6.
[http://dx.doi.org/10.4258/hir.2010.16.1.65] [PMID: 22509475]

CHAPTER 6

Innovative Payment Models and Financial Technology in Healthcare

Akhil Sharma[1], Ashish Verma[2], Akanksha Sharma[1], Sunita[1], Neeraj Kumar Fuloria[3] and Shaweta Sharma[4,*]

[1] *R.J. College of Pharmacy, Raipur, Gharbara, Tappal, Khair, Uttar Pradesh 202165, India*

[2] *Mangalmay Pharmacy College, Greater Noida, Uttar Pradesh 201306, India*

[3] *Department of Pharmaceutical Chemistry, Faculty of Pharmacy, AIMST University, Semeling Campus, Jalan Bedong-Semeling 08100 Bedong, Kedah Darul Aman, Malaysia*

[4] *School of Medical and Allied Sciences, Galgotias University, Yamuna Expressway, Gautam Buddha Nagar, Uttar Pradesh 201310, India*

Abstract: Traditional healthcare payment systems have led to escalating costs, inefficiencies, and inequities in access to care, underscoring the need for payment innovation, adoption of financial technologies (FinTech), and collaborative efforts to establish an efficient, accessible, and sustainable healthcare ecosystem. This chapter examines the transition in healthcare financing via value-based payment designs, digital payment systems, and financial technology. When healthcare systems adopt value-based care instead of fee-for-service, they recognise the importance of outcomes over volume and employ models such as bundled payments, accountable care organisations, and capitation to improve care delivery while controlling costs. The financial technology sector revolutionises the payment process with greater transparency, reduced administrative load, and increased accessibility. Tech advancements in FinTech, like mobile wallets and blockchain, enable safe transactions and facilitate microloans and predictive analytics using AI that helps with payment, resource optimisation, and improved financial accessibility for the unbanked. It also explores how InsurTech solutions like automated claims processing and usage-based insurance models are helping to align financial incentives with patient outcomes better. The sustainability of financial expenditure through technology services to reduce cost, improve efficiency, and resource optimisation is a crucial focus area. Examples from worldwide healthcare systems reveal practical applications of innovative payment models and FinTech solutions that can improve affordability and financial stability. The chapter ends with advice on overcoming barriers to adoption, dealing with regulatory issues, and promoting stakeholder cooperation. Innovative payment models

* **Corresponding author Shaweta Sharma:** School of Medical and Allied Sciences, Galgotias University, Yamuna Expressway, Gautam Buddha Nagar, Uttar Pradesh 201310, India; E-mail: shawetasharma@galgotiasuniversity.edu.in

and FinTech, if harnessed by healthcare systems, can lead to optimised delivery and uniform access, along with greenhouse gas emissions, ultimately resulting in long-term sustainability.

Keywords: Digital payment solutions, Financial technology (fintech), Financial sustainability, Healthcare financing, Innovative payment models, Resource allocation, Value-based care.

INTRODUCTION

Payment models in healthcare also include the different types of frameworks and strategies used for reimbursement for the services provided by the healthcare provider to the patient. These models dictate the transactions between payers, such as government agencies and insurance companies, and patient providers, including hospitals, clinics, and individual practitioners. Fee-for-service or other traditional models reimburse providers for each separate service or procedure, thereby encouraging volume over value. In contrast, newer payment models, such as value-based care, focus on quality, patient outcomes, and cost-effectiveness. These frameworks look to align economic incentives with the provision of appropriate, patient-centric care while addressing waste in the use of resources and financial viability. Models of payment significantly affect how the healthcare system is structured, notably in terms of access, affordability, and the type of care patients receive [1 - 8].

Revolutionising the financial aspect of healthcare, FinTech is also trying to facilitate payments between organisations more efficiently, with mobile wallets, online payments, and blockchain technology, both of which streamline transactions whilst needing less administration and encouraging secure, on-time reimbursements. It widens financial access with devices like microloans and crowdfunding, making treatments affordable for patients.

Importance of Financial Sustainability in Healthcare Systems

Financial sustainability allows for consistently implementing quality healthcare and accommodating growing populations in evolving sectors requiring health protection, prevention and care. The sustainability of finance enables healthcare organisations to be resource-pooled, allowing for higher efficiency in operations while also facilitating investment of healthcare systems in infrastructure development, including workforce development and innovative technologies. Such stability ensures fair access to medical services, especially with limited resources, and hospitals tend to be oversaturated [9, 10].

In addition, it enables long-term planning for healthcare systems to address emerging pressures such as the increasing costs of complex therapies, changes in demographics, and global health crises. This means public health programs such as vaccinations, preventive care, and chronic disease management can function without interruption. To governments and policymakers, financing is sustainable when it is less dependent on external funding sources and minimises the pressure that can propagate through sectors, thus better distributing resources [11, 12].

Moreover, financial sustainability attracts investments and creates space for innovation in the private sector by establishing a stable and predictable business environment. It allows stakeholders to partner to generate cost-effective solutions and develop new healthcare delivery models. Additionally, sustainability directly impacts patient satisfaction and outcomes as financially sustainable systems can prioritise affordability and accessibility alongside high-quality care [13, 14].

Financial sustainability is achievable through progressive payment mechanisms, utilisation of financial technology tools, and efforts at cost containment amidst escalating healthcare costs. It is a pillar of resilient healthcare systems that can respond to change and maintain vital services to populations on all continents [15].

CHALLENGES IN TRADITIONAL PAYMENT MODELS IN HEALTHCARE

The challenges that occur in traditional payment models in healthcare are described below and summarised in Fig. (1).

Fee-for-Service Models and Rising Costs

The Fee-for-Service (FFS) model is a longstanding form of payment in healthcare that compensates providers for services or procedures rendered. This model rewards prompt and predictable compensation for each clinical intervention but inherently promotes quantity over quality. Financial incentives drive healthcare providers to perform more services, which results in unnecessary tests, procedures, and treatments regardless of their clinical needs [16, 17]. This leads to increased healthcare costs as healthcare providers provide services that may not lead to better outcomes for the patient. Patients are often left with rising medical bills as they are provided services, and bills upon bills mount into even for routine care and high out-of-pocket expenses. Increasing costs of FFS models and complaints about administrative inefficiencies have prompted calls for alternative, value-based care models that prioritise patient outcomes over the volume of services provided [18, 19].

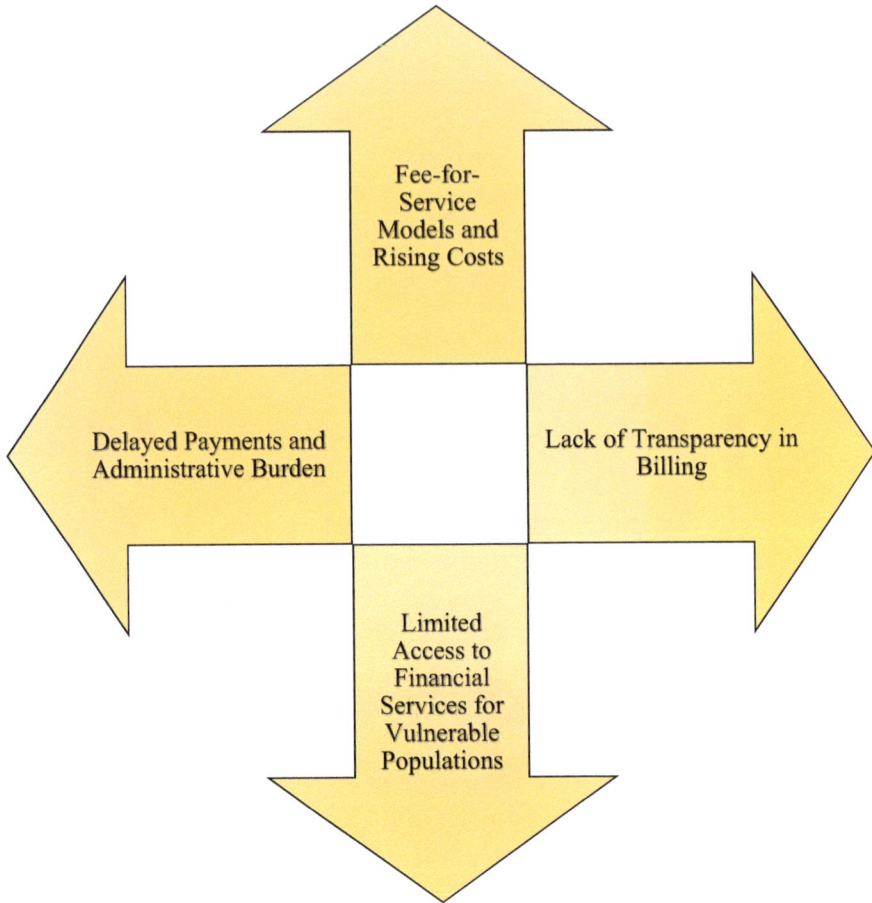

Fig. (1). Challenges in traditional payment models in healthcare.

Delayed Payments and Administrative Burden

Traditional payment systems are often slow and unwieldy, with billings from insurers or government programs taking weeks or months to process. This delay can cause serious cash flow issues, particularly for smaller practices or those in rural areas. Meanwhile, providers who rely on timely reimbursement must try to manage operational costs and the wages of the staff who care for their residents without them [20, 21]. The traditional billing system is also highly complex, with a significant administrative burden in tracking claims, fighting with insurers, and ensuring compliance with frequently changing rules. These administrative costs take away resources from patient care and can lead to increased healthcare costs. The delays negatively impact providers and patients, who often wait for payments to keep their operations afloat [22, 23].

Lack of Transparency in Billing

The lack of billing transparency is one of the biggest detriments of traditional payment models. Pricing could differ significantly between FFS providers for the same procedures or services. Patients can be socked with surprise bills because of hidden fees or confusion around what's billed to insurance versus what patients owe out-of-pocket. So many different billing codes and the fact that they cannot compare costs across healthcare providers have made it difficult for patients to understand the costs of care they receive [24, 25]. Without price transparency, patients lack the information necessary to make informed healthcare decisions, often finding out the full price only after that care has been delivered. It also exposes patients to surprise medical bills, especially when they receive out-of-network care, further increasing financial distress and eroding trust in the healthcare system [26, 27].

Limited Access to Financial Services for Vulnerable Populations

The fee-for-service payment system cannot address the needs of the most vulnerable populations, who often miss out on care due to the financial burden it imposes. These include low-income people, the uninsured, and those without access to credit or financial services. Because many of these people cannot afford to pay in full for medical services upfront or have insured claims with high out-of-pocket amounts, they become the debtors for a service they cannot afford. Even with insurance, the high deductibles and copayments mean many others cannot afford health care [28, 29].

In addition, lower-income people typically have no access to financial products that could make it easier to cover medical bills, like payment plans, lines of credit or health savings accounts. Without such tools, this group may hesitate to pursue necessary care, resulting in poorer health outcomes over the longer term. It also contributes to healthcare inequalities, wherein patients from lower socioeconomic status regions encounter extra hurdles when getting adequate medical help or medicines owing to financial constraints [30, 31].

EMERGING PAYMENT MODELS IN HEALTHCARE

Value-Based Payment Models

Value-based payment models shift reimbursement from a volume-based system for services into a model that ties the reimbursement to the quality of the care delivered. The goal is to encourage healthcare providers to improve patient outcomes while reducing costs. These models promote coordinated, patient-centred care that values health outcomes over the volume of treatments or procedures [32]. Below are some kcy types of value-based payment models:

Pay-for-Performance (P4P)

Pay-for-performance (P4P) is a value-based payment model in which healthcare providers are rewarded for attaining certain quality and performance targets. In this framework, healthcare providers are provided with motivation to meet pre-established quality metrics; these metrics can include improving patient satisfaction, reducing readmission rates, or complying with clinical guidelines [33, 34]. Providers can earn financial incentives for achieving these goals and face decreased payments or penalties if they do not perform well against performance metrics. The purpose of P4P is to incentivise the delivery of high-quality care and eliminate waste and error in the healthcare system. One challenge, however, is that metrics must be carefully crafted to be achievable and equitable and to measure quality care [35, 36].

Bundled Payments

In bundled payments, a single, fixed payment covers a related group of healthcare services delivered over time. Rather than compensating providers separately for each service (*e.g.,* doctor visits, hospital stays, and surgeries), a bundled payment covers the entire episode of care. A relevant example is a bundled payment for all things related to knee replacement surgery, including pre-operative assessment, surgery and post-operative rehabilitation [37, 38].

The mission is to motivate providers to collaborate more efficiently and cost-effectively and minimise unnecessary procedures or hospital readmissions. Because they are jointly accountable for the total cost of care for the patient, bundled payments encourage better coordination among multiple care providers. However, the main challenge of this model is how to make all providers, including specialists, work together under the payment bundle to prevent fragmentation of care or gaps in service delivery [39, 40].

Accountable Care Organizations (ACOs)

Accountable Care Organizations (ACOs) comprise a group of healthcare providers, such as hospitals, doctors, and other clinicians, collaborating to deliver healthcare services to a target patient population. The ACO is ultimately responsible for the quality of care provided to its patients and their total cost of care. The benefits of shared savings, where ACOs can earn a percentage of the savings achieved through improved quality, cost control, and patient satisfaction compared to a shared target, only occur if they meet a particular set of process and outcome performance measures [41, 42]. ACOs aim to eliminate unnecessary tests, reduce hospital readmissions, and enhance preventive care. A key issue related to ACOs comes from the increased complexity of managing this care across many organisations and ensuring communication and planning among providers, especially as patient needs become more complex [43, 44].

Capitation and Global Budgets

Capitation and global budgets are alternative payment models in which healthcare providers are given a fixed amount of money per patient per year, regardless of how many services the patient receives. These models are designed to encourage providers to deliver preventive care and avoid unnecessary services because they must cover the cost of care in its entirety [45].

Capitation

With capitation, healthcare providers receive a fixed amount per patient at a flat rate. They are paid usually each month or at least once per year, including any necessary treatment, ranging from hospital visits to physician consultations, medication, and so on. The fixed payment is intended to address the complete healthcare needs of an entire population. In a capitated system, the healthcare provider is paid a fixed rate per patient, incentivising them to provide the most effective and cost-efficient care possible. At the same time, providers may restrict access to essential services or avoid high-risk patients to increase their profits [46, 47].

Global Budgets

Global budgets are similar to capitation but are generally applied to entire healthcare organisations (for instance, a hospital or a health plan) or systems rather than individual providers. A global budget allocates a set amount of funding for all healthcare services delivered to a population or over a defined period. Such systems or organisations have to allocate financial resources wisely to address the health needs of their population [48, 49]. This approach aims to enhance care coordination, eliminate unnecessary spending, and provide resources for preventive and primary care services, which can help avoid costly interventions. However, global budgets may face challenges in adjusting to unpredictable fluctuations in patient needs or emergencies, and there may be concerns about quality if providers are overly focused on reducing costs [50, 51].

Outcome-Based Payment Models

Outcome-based payment models (pay-for-outcomes) emphasise linking reimbursement to the clinical outcomes achieved by care. Instead of chasing the volume of services provided, these models focus on the quality of patient outcomes, such as recovery rates, functional improvements, or long-term health conditions management. This encourages healthcare providers to provide care that ultimately leads to better patient health outcomes and enhances the healthcare system's overall effectiveness [52].

With outcome-based models, the uses of clinical benchmarks and metrics of provider performance data are shared. For instance, a healthcare provider might be incentivised to meet specific targets for improved patient health, including mortality reduction and quality of life for chronic disease patients [53]. One of the areas where it is frequently applied in chronic disease management or preventive care is where the successful management of chronic conditions such as diabetes, hypertension, or heart disease can be linked to financial incentives. However, a challenge with this model is accurately evaluating patient outcomes and considering different factors (such as patient demographics and socio-economic factors) to avoid penalising healthcare providers who treat high-risk populations. Moreover, the correct incentive mechanics of the models must be substantiated using advanced data analytics monitoring outcomes [54, 55].

ROLE OF FINANCIAL TECHNOLOGY (FINTECH) IN HEALTHCARE

FinTech is a rapidly growing sector making inroads into various industries, including healthcare. FinTech is improving healthcare efficiency, accessibility, and affordability through digital payment solutions, patient financing tools, insurance technology, and artificial intelligence [56, 57]. Below are the key areas where FinTech is making an impact, also depicted in Fig. (**2**).

Digital Payment Solutions

Digital payment solutions are transforming the patient payment experience. Many mobile wallets and online payment systems make it easy for patients to pay their medical bills through smartphones or computers. Since it lowers the administrative load, it makes payment convenient for the patient and the medical staff, as they do not have to carry cash or cheques to make payments [58, 59]. Moreover, blockchain technology is applied to secure transactions within the healthcare ecosystem. However, blockchain can help prevent fraud by providing a decentralised ledger that ensures transparency and security, preventing unauthorised access to sensitive financial information. This payment security framework, trusted by patients and providers alike, normalises payment most efficiently while guaranteeing secure transactions of funds [60, 61].

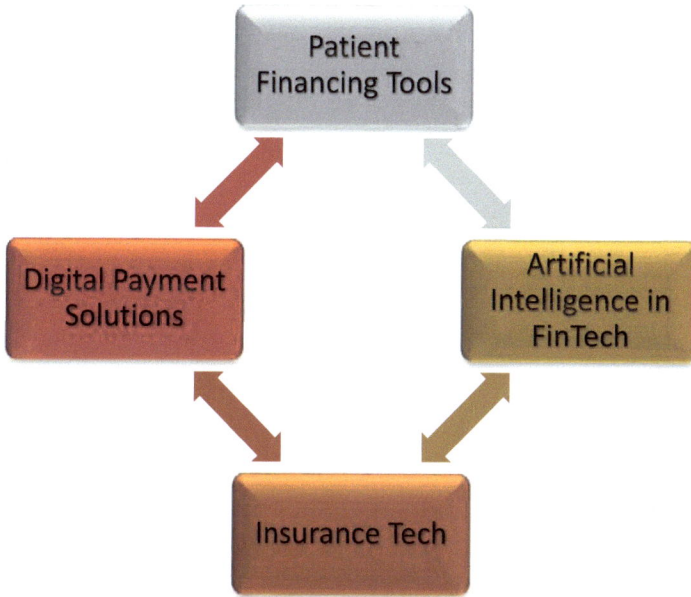

Fig. (2). Role of financial technology (fintech) in healthcare.

Patient Financing Tools

Patient financing tools are the key to triaging the high out-of-pocket costs associated with healthcare. Healthcare microloans refer to understanding and providing a small loan tailored for the healthcare sector to help patients overcome medical expenses by allowing them to receive necessary treatments without incurring immediate financial burdens. These loans frequently offer adaptable payment solutions customised to individual situations, allowing individuals to access healthcare without putting off or avoiding treatment altogether due to money concerns [62, 63]. Such platforms were also an option for patients seeking help with medical expenses. These platforms enable individuals to gather money from friends, family and the wider community to cover the costs of surgeries, treatments or emergencies. Crowdfunding harnesses the ability of social networks and online communities to provide alternative funding sources to relieve the financial burden on patients and their families [64, 65].

Insurance Tech

Insurance technology (InsurTech) is revolutionising health insurance by automating claims processing and establishing new insurance models. Automated claims processing enables insurance claims to be submitted and approved in less time and with less effort required of healthcare providers and patients. Insurance companies need to move digitally and integrated with EHR (electronic health records) because this digital solution will make the insurance claim process much faster with minimum errors and reimbursements [66, 67]. This automation, in addition to optimising cash for healthcare providers, improves the patient experience by generating fewer delays in claims approvals. In addition, usage-based insurance models are being adopted in the healthcare industry. This leads to premiums being charged based on usage of the services rather than being fixed, so that patients who do not need a lot of medical care can afford insurance. These approaches encourage fairness and accessibility in health insurance by linking costs to the actual use of health care [68, 69].

Artificial Intelligence in FinTech

AI is revolutionising FinTech applications in healthcare, especially for fraud prevention and predictive analytics in cost optimisation. They use a large amount of transaction data for analysis and pattern analysis using AI fraud detection systems to spot unusual patterns or anomalies for potential fraudulent activities. Machine learning algorithms enhance these systems' accuracy over time, reducing the risk of financial losses through fraud for patients and healthcare providers [70, 71]. By analysing historical data and trends, AI-enabled predictive analytics can predict and optimise future healthcare costs. By analysing parameters like patient demographics, treatment history, and regional healthcare costs, AI can help organisations anticipate financial needs and allocate resources accordingly. By taking this proactive approach, healthcare organisations can better budget and manage their financial resources, ultimately improving patient care outcomes [72, 73].

FINANCIAL EXPENDITURE SUSTAINABILITY

Financial expenditure sustainability refers to an organisation's, government's, or entity's ability to manage its financial resources effectively to ensure that current and future expenditures can be met without compromising financial stability or operational capacity. This concept is crucial for maintaining long-term viability and involves strategic planning, responsible budgeting, and effective resource allocation.

Components of Financial Expenditure Sustainability

Revenue Generation

A predictable revenue stream is needed to ensure sustainable expenditures. Strategies that drive multiple sources of revenue must sit at the top of this list if organisations want to maintain the ability to pay the bills. Organisations should consider diversifying their income, including taxes, grants, donations, service fees, and investments, since relying on one form of revenue can be risky. An example would be non-profit organisations applying for grants from foundations and government organisations and doing fundraisers to increase the organisation's income sources. At the same time, companies can boost revenues by investing in activities that drive economic expansion, including investing in new goods or products or new sectors. Long-term contracts with clients or partners also provide a revenue stream to ensure the continued availability of maintenance and operations funding [74, 75].

Cost Management

Expenditure management is a must for financial sustainability. Organisations should analyse and control operational expenditure to avoid over-expenditure and ensure proper allocation of resources. Adopting a strict budgeting process helps organisations channel essential spending and identify areas to cut costs. Strategies like zero-based budgeting demand the rationale behind every outlay to be established anew every cycle, fostering a culture of responsibility and optimising resource utilisation [76, 77]. Monitoring expenses versus budget regularly allows organisations to catch variances and flag overspending early; financial software facilitates this process with up-to-date visibility of spending patterns. Additionally, companies must explore avenues to enhance operational efficiency by optimising processes and leveraging technologies, employing lean management principles for waste reduction and workflow optimisation [78].

Long-term Financial Planning

Planning for the long and short term is essential in foreseeing future needs and expectations. Organisations should rely on comprehensive forecasting based on historical data and overarching business goals to draw a line of sight of where the business wants to go financially. Methods like forecasting techniques, including trend or regression analysis and scenario planning, allow organisations to anticipate future revenues and expenses. This aids in identifying potential financial difficulties sooner rather than later. Financial strategies should also address long-range plans to ensure that decision-making continues to be aligned with the organisation's strategic goals and that human and financial resources are aligned with the overall goals of the mission objectives. Strategic investments in such areas are equally important; organisations must ensure that new projects or equipment purchases provide a solid return on investment (ROI) that supports long-term sustainability [79, 80].

Risk Management

Detecting and mitigating monetary dangers is crucial to highlight the sustainability of expenses. They should evaluate risks that may arise, including recession, policy changes, or unexpected costs, and prepare for this by developing contingency plans. By doing regular audits of returns or assessing the risk through risk assessment tools, a structured risk assessment framework helps recognise the vulnerability of an organisation's financial operation. Contingency planning involves preparing for unforeseen circumstances affecting finances, such as setting up emergency accounts or credit lines that can be drawn upon when disaster strikes. Businesses are better protected from unexpected liabilities and losses through sufficient insurance coverage; undertaking routine assessments of insurance policies helps guarantee that current risks and organisational needs are being met through coverage [81, 82].

Performance Measurement

Financial performance, measured and compared against benchmarks regularly, is critical to any sustainability assessment. Financial organisations must track their effectiveness based on key performance indicators (KPIs) like revenue growth, expense control, and overall economic health. KPIs should be relevant to the organisation and its goals, but typical KPIs include operating margin, return on assets (ROA), liquidity ratios, and cost per service unit delivered. Employing data analytics tools augments the ability to track performance metrics; graphical representations of essential financial variables permit decision-makers to rapidly evaluate the economic status of the enterprise and make adjustments as warranted. Lastly, the performance measurement process must generate insights that inform action items directed towards improving various aspects of an organisation; routine performance reporting can help identify gaps which require attention or strategic repositioning [83, 84].

Working on Financial Expenditure Sustainability

Financial expenditure sustainability operates through a structured cycle of planning, execution, monitoring, and adjustment. Each phase is crucial for ensuring an organisation can effectively manage its financial resources over the long term while adapting to changing circumstances and needs [85]. The working of financial expenditure sustainability is summarised in Fig. (**3**).

Planning

The planning phase is the backbone of sustainable financial expenditure, as it comprises preparing comprehensive budgets detailing anticipated revenues and expenses over a specified period. This involves gathering input from department heads, financial officers, and external advisors to ensure the budget aligns with the organisation's strategic goals. In this process, organisations examine the realities of their current financial position, past spending behaviours, and anticipated accrual of income. In addition to these internal challenges, they must navigate external factors, including economic trends, regulatory changes, and market conditions that influence financial performance. An organised budget is a financial roadmap that allows flexibility to adapt to unforeseen costs or revenue fluctuations. Organisations may also establish specific financial targets in this stage, for example, a percentage decrease in costs or an increase in income from particular programs, which inform decision-making throughout the budgeting process [86].

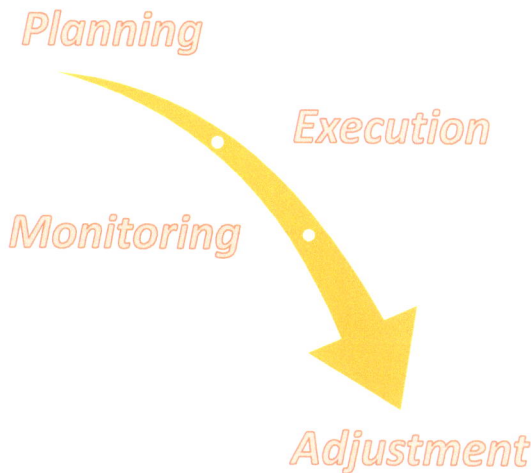

Fig. (3). Working of financial expenditure sustainability.

Execution

The execution phase occurs after the budget is set, where plans are executed by assigning resources in alignment with the approved budget. They must focus on balancing all levels of everyday expenditures with what is available within the budget limitation, yet accomplish the mission by utilising resources most directly and advantageously as possible. This means both organisations must inform each department and the individual staff members how the budget will work in practice, including what they can and cannot do regarding expenditure. This could include training sessions or workshops that help employees understand how to work with new processes or tools for budgeting and resource allocation. Additionally, organisations need to implement internal controls to track spending against their budget in real-time so they are aware of any discrepancies or potential overspending as it is happening. Successful implementation is also about fostering accountability where budgets are handled proactively at the department level, with an eye towards a more excellent organisation [87, 88].

Monitoring

Budget monitoring is vital to determine any deviations from the budget and whether an entity is on course to meet its spending objectives. This phase includes frequent checks of financial reports and a set of KPIs, which help the company see how the revenue is generated and spent. Organisations usually employ financial management software that enables real-time monitoring of outflows relative to the budget to identify trends and outliers swiftly. Regular meetings with department heads can initiate a conversation about how their budget is performing and what obstacles were faced in this plan. Monitoring should not simply be about spotting what is going wrong but also what is going right, where departments may be exceeding expectations or saving money—this continuous conversation about financial performance positions organisations to adjust proactively rather than reactively [89, 90].

Adjustment

Organisations must modify their budget or operational plan to ensure continued sustainability based on their monitoring results. The cornerstone for success in this innovation process is the adjustment period, determining how to adapt to changes in various parameters, such as unforeseen spending, revenue stream fluctuations, or changing strategic priorities. Organisations should have established guidelines for making changes, including reallocating resources from failed initiatives to cutting unnecessary expenses identified during monitoring. Moreover, organisations can pursue entrepreneurial revenue streams that will support the diversification of funding sources or expand successful programs. Discussing what the organisation needs to change with stakeholders creates transparency and encourages collaboration and progress. This adaptive approach steers organisations towards resilience amidst challenges while keeping their long-term financial sustainability at the forefront [91, 92].

CASE STUDIES

By highlighting successful implementations, case studies showcase the transformative potential of novel financial models in healthcare. Value-based care models have been successful at improving patient outcomes and controlling costs. As an illustration, implementing Pay-for-Performance (P4P) programs in the U.S. has encouraged hospitals and doctors to provide high-quality care, resulting in better patient satisfaction and lower hospital readmission rates. Meanwhile, Accountable Care Organizations (ACOs) have also shown effective care coordination across providers, leading to lower care costs due to the prevention of avoidable treatments and hospital admissions [93].

Blockchain has revolutionised transparent billing. These findings have led to the increasing adoption of blockchain by hospitals and insurers alike, simplifying their billing processes, increasing transparency, and lowering instances of fraud. Blockchain generates a secure and unchangeable record of transactions that allows patients to follow healthcare spending similar to that of a credit card, allowing for accuracy and accountability regarding financial exchanges [94].

FinTech startups are making a big difference. Companies such as OakNorth and Cedar are leveraging technology to provide more efficient payment platforms, easing the friction between patients, providers, and insurers. Such platforms offer technology-driven solutions such as AI-driven billing systems and mobile wallet integration, further streamlining the payment process and allowing patients easier access to paying bills (especially those in underserved areas). Their disruptive models are helping to reduce administrative costs and improve overall financial sustainability within healthcare systems. Together, these case studies reflect the potential for financial technology to reshape healthcare payment structures and ensure long-term sustainability [95].

BARRIERS TO THE ADOPTION OF INNOVATIVE PAYMENT MODELS

The integration of novel payment models into healthcare delivery continues to encounter barriers that slow the uptake of these new models. Regulations and compliance issues are the most significant barriers, as existing healthcare regulations may not be flexible enough to align with new payment systems such as value-based care or outcome-based models. Healthcare systems must navigate complex legal requirements and ensure that any new models comply with national and regional laws, which can slow down the adoption process. Moreover, barriers to interoperability in financial systems are a fundamental challenge [96].

Different healthcare providers, insurance companies, and financial institutions typically have different technology platforms, which makes it hard to share information and process payments seamlessly. Without sound systems for integration and smooth movement of information, the efficiency of novel payment models can be compromised. Resistance from major stakeholders like patients, providers, and insurers also adds to the challenge of moving to new payment methods. Many healthcare professionals may be reluctant to adopt new models amidst fears about reimbursement rates, administrative burden or long-term financial viability [97].

On the other hand, patients may be wary of changes to their out-of-pocket costs or access to care. Finally, low-resource settings experience technology gaps that make implementing advanced payment models even more challenging. Providers in less developed regions may be unable to adopt and maintain digital payment solutions or data-sharing systems, further impairing the possibility of broad execution in these regions. This collectively highlights the importance of careful planning and tailored strategies to ensure a successful transition to more efficient, equitable healthcare payment systems [98].

FUTURE DIRECTIONS

Advanced technologies like AI (Artificial Intelligence) and ML (Machine Learning) in FinTech have a significant amount of potential for improving the efficiency of numerous financial transactions and decision-making processes, which in the coming years and decades will shape payment models of healthcare. AI and ML streamline claims processing, anticipate patient needs, and fine-tune reimbursement rates, thus minimising costs while maximising patient health outcomes [99, 100].

Another priority area is broadening healthcare access in rural and underserved environments that often lack financial instruments and optimal healthcare services. Mobile technologies, microloans, and telehealth platforms can help fill these gaps and ensure that underserved populations can access the necessary healthcare services and financing options. Further, policy recommendations will be needed to promote the uptake of new payment models. Governments can be essential influencers by developing regulatory frameworks that support value-based care, bundled payments and other alternative models while ensuring compliance requirements do not stifle innovation [101].

Finally, public-private partnerships (PPPs) have immense potential to transform healthcare finance by pooling resources, expertise, and technologies. These partnerships can facilitate the adoption of infrastructure, fund pilot programs, and scale successful paradigms, driving sustainability and efficiency in global health systems. These developments suggest a future where healthcare payment systems are more adaptive, fair, and sustainable, leading to greater access and quality of care [102].

CONCLUSION

Integrating FinTech in healthcare payments can bring a considerable change in the whole system with access, affordability, and efficiency improvements. FinTech enhances financial transactions, lowers administrative burdens, and guarantees speedy payments through digital payment, patient financing solutions, and process automation. Transitioning to advanced payment models like value-based care and AI-driven predictive analytics enables better resource allocation, cost control, and financial sustainability. As the healthcare landscape continues to evolve, FinTech's role in ensuring the sustainability of financial expenditure becomes increasingly essential, providing tools for better cost management and decision-making. By reducing financial barriers and increasing transparency, FinTech fosters a more equitable healthcare system, broadening access to treatment, particularly in these underserved regions, and improving overall patient outcomes. A sustainable and efficient new healthcare system will depend on the successful integration of innovative payment models and the effective use of technology to consolidate and minimise deeply bureaucratically intertwined financial processes, enabling affordable quality healthcare for all.

CONSENT FOR PUBLICATON

All authors have given their consent for publication. The authors authorised Dr. Shaweta Sharma to handle all correspondences.

ACKNOWLEDGEMENTS

Authors are highly thankful to their Universities/Colleges for providing library facilities for the literature survey.

REFERENCES

[1]   Thompson KK. Aligning payment with quality. Am J Health Syst Pharm 2008; 65(16): 1512.
      [http://dx.doi.org/10.2146/ajhp080274] [PMID: 18693204]

[2]   Jia L, Meng Q, Scott A, Yuan B, Zhang L. Payment methods for healthcare providers working in outpatient healthcare settings. Cochrane Database Syst Rev 2021; 1(1): CD011865

[3]   Crowley R, Daniel H, Cooney TG, Engel LS, Health and public policy committee of the American college of physicians. Envisioning a better U.S. health care system for all: coverage and cost of care. Ann Intern Med. 2020; 172 (2 Suppl): S7-S32.
      [http://dx.doi.org/10.7326/M19-2415] [PMID: 31958805]

[4]   Schoen C, Osborn R, Squires D, Doty MM, Pierson R, Applebaum S. How health insurance design affects access to care and costs, by income, in eleven countries. Health Aff (Millwood) 2010; 29(12): 2323-34.
      [http://dx.doi.org/10.1377/hlthaff.2010.0862] [PMID: 21088012]

[5]   Cambaza E. The role of fintech in sustainable healthcare development in sub-Saharan Africa: a narrative review. FinTech 2023; 2(3): 444-60.
      [http://dx.doi.org/10.3390/fintech2030025]

[6]   Babu SK, et al. Analyzing the digital transformation and evolution of financial technology (fintech) across various industries. In: 2024 4th International Conference on Innovative Practices in Technology and Management (ICIPTM) Noida, India: IEEE 2024; pp. 1–8.

[7]   Tsevat J, Moriates C. Value-based health care meets cost-effectiveness analysis. Ann Intern Med 2018; 169(5): 329-32.
      [http://dx.doi.org/10.7326/M18-0342] [PMID: 30083766]

[8]   McClellan M. Reforming payments to healthcare providers: the key to slowing healthcare cost growth while improving quality? J Econ Perspect 2011; 25(2): 69-92.
[http://dx.doi.org/10.1257/jep.25.2.69] [PMID: 21595326]

[9]   Liaropoulos L, Goranitis I. Health care financing and the sustainability of health systems. Int J Equity Health 2015; 14(1): 80.
[http://dx.doi.org/10.1186/s12939-015-0208-5] [PMID: 26369417]

[10]   Deshkukh B, Waghamare S. Medical tourism in India: Challenges and opportunities. ACADEMICIA: An Intl Multidis Res J 2021; 11(3): 2288-99.
[http://dx.doi.org/10.5958/2249-7137.2021.01003.X]

[11]   Valieva EN, Yarullin RR, Zhelonkin NN, Mayorskaya AS. Innovations in financial sustainability management of public health care organisations. In: Ashmarina SI, Mantulenko VV, Vochozka M, Eds. Engineering economics: decisions and solutions from Eurasian perspective. Cham: Springer International Publishing 2021; pp. 191–200.

[12]   Abbasi WA, Wang Z, Abbasi DA. Potential sources of financing for small and medium enterprises (SMEs) and the role of government in supporting SMEs. J Small Bus Entrep Dev 2017; 5(2): 39-47.

[13]   Carmo Filho RD, Borges PP. Financial management, efficiency, and care quality: A systematic review in the context of Health 4.0. Health services management research. 2025 May; 38(2): 107-19.
[http://dx.doi.org/10.1177/09514848241275783]

[14]   Tetteh PA, Osei-Kyei R, Tam VW. Strategies for sustainable financing of circular infrastructure projects–a systematic review. Construction Innovation 2025 Jun 5; 25(7): 235-67.
[http://dx.doi.org/10.1108/CI-10-2024-032]

[15]   Kilci EN. A study on financial sustainability of healthcare indicators for Turkey under the health transformation program. Int J Health Plann Manage 2021; 36(4): 1287-307.
[http://dx.doi.org/10.1002/hpm.3182] [PMID: 33884667]

[16]   Conquest JH, Gill N, Sivanujan P, Skinner J, Kruger E, Tennant M. Systematic literature review of capitation and fee-for-service payment models for oral health services: an Australian perspective. Healthcare 2021; 9(9): 1129.
[http://dx.doi.org/10.3390/healthcare9091129]

[17]   Ginsburg PB. Fee-for-service will remain a feature of major payment reforms, requiring more changes in Medicare physician payment. Health Aff (Millwood) 2012; 31(9): 1977-83.
[http://dx.doi.org/10.1377/hlthaff.2012.0350] [PMID: 22949446]

[18]   Hoffman AK, Jackson HE. Retiree out-of-pocket healthcare spending: a study of consumer expectations and policy implications. Am J Law Med 2013; 39(1): 62-133.
[http://dx.doi.org/10.1177/009885881303900102] [PMID: 23678788]

[19]   Edmiston KD. Alternative payment models, value-based payments, and health disparities. Center for Insurance Policy & Research Report at the National Association of Insurance Commissioners. 2022: 1-47.
[http://dx.doi.org/10.52227/25526.2022]

[20]   Hankede M, Mwelwa A. Assessing the Factors Causing Delay by Insurance Companies to Pay Claims to Customers: A case of selected Insurance Companies, and Pensions and Insurance Authority (PIA). East Afri Fin J 2024; 3(2): 234-61.
[http://dx.doi.org/10.59413/eafj/v3.i2.8]

[21]   Lemma S. Factors affecting motor insurance claim processing time: the case of Awash Insurance Company SC. PhD dissertation. Addis Ababa (Ethiopia): St. Mary's University 2019.

[22]   Bazel MA, Mohammed F, Ahmed M. Blockchain technology in healthcare big data management: benefits, applications and challenges. In: Proceedings of the 2021 1st International Conference on Emerging Smart Technologies and Applications (eSmarTA); 2021 Aug 10; Sana'a, Yemen. Piscataway (NJ): IEEE 2021; pp. 1–8.

[23] Cutler DM. Reducing administrative costs in US health care. Hamilton Project Policy Proposal 2020; 9: 3-25.

[24] Chen J, Miraldo M. The impact of hospital price and quality transparency tools on healthcare spending: a systematic review. Health Econ Rev 2022; 12(1): 62.
[http://dx.doi.org/10.1186/s13561-022-00409-4] [PMID: 36515792]

[25] Hilsenrath P, Eakin C, Fischer K. Price-transparency and cost accounting: challenges for health care organizations in the consumer-driven era. Inquiry 2015; 52: 0046958015574981.
[http://dx.doi.org/10.1177/0046958015574981] [PMID: 25862425]

[26] Reed RD. Costs and benefits: Price transparency in health care. J Health Care Finance 2019.

[27] Long C, Cho BH, Giladi AM. Understanding surprise out-of-network billing in hand and upper extremity care. J Hand Surg Am 2021; 46(3): 236-40.
[http://dx.doi.org/10.1016/j.jhsa.2020.11.008] [PMID: 33358882]

[28] Shrank WH, DeParle NA, Gottlieb S, *et al.* Health Costs And Financing: Challenges And Strategies For A New Administration: Commentary recommends health cost, financing, and other priorities for a new US administration. Health Aff (Millwood) 2021; 40(2): 235-42.
[http://dx.doi.org/10.1377/hlthaff.2020.01560]

[29] Dawkins B, Renwick C, Ensor T, Shinkins B, Jayne D, Meads D. What factors affect patients' healthcare access? An overview of systematic reviews. Trop Med Int Health 2021; 26(10): 1177-88.
[http://dx.doi.org/10.1111/tmi.13651] [PMID: 34219346]

[30] Harper A, Staeheli M, Edwards D, Herring Y, Baker M. Disabled, poor, and poorly served: Access to and use of financial services by people with serious mental illness. Soc Serv Rev 2018; 92(2): 202-40.
[http://dx.doi.org/10.1086/697904]

[31] Betancourt JR, Maina A. Betancourt JR, Maina A Barriers to eliminating disparities in clinical practice: lessons from the IOM report "Unequal Treatment" In: Smedley BD, Stith AY, Nelson AR, Eds Eliminating healthcare disparities in America: beyond the IOM report Totowa (NJ): Humana Press 2007 pp 83–97. Totowa, NJ: Humana Press 2007; pp. 83-97.

[32] Leao DL, Cremers HP, van Veghel D, Pavlova M, Groot W. The impact of Value-based payment models for Care and Transmural Care networks: a systematic literature review. Appl Health Econ Health Policy 2023; 21(3): 441-66.
[http://dx.doi.org/10.1007/s40258-023-00790-z] [PMID: 36723777]

[33] Yu ZA, Gorgone MB. Pay-for-performance and value-based care. Treasure Island (FL): StatPearls Publishing 2025

[34] Sura A, Shah NR. Pay-for-performance initiatives: modest benefits for improving healthcare quality. Am Health Drug Benefits 2010; 3(2): 135-42.
[PMID: 25126315]

[35] Greene SE, Nash DB. Pay for performance: an overview of the literature. Am J Med Qual 2009; 24(2): 140-63.
[http://dx.doi.org/10.1177/1062860608326517] [PMID: 18984907]

[36] Slawomirski L, Hensher M, Campbell J, deGraaff B. Pay-for-performance and patient safety in acute care: A systematic review. Health Policy 2024; 143: 105051.
[http://dx.doi.org/10.1016/j.healthpol.2024.105051] [PMID: 38547664]

[37] Agyemang CO, Boakye RA, Gyamfi G. Leveraging health data analytics to drive inclusive Medicaid expansion and immigrant healthcare policy reform. Int J Comput Appl Technol Res 2025; 14(6) :1-8.
[http://dx.doi.org/10.7753/IJCATR1406.1001]

[38] Adida E, Mamani H, Nassiri S. Bundled payment vs. fee-for-service: Impact of payment scheme on performance. Manage Sci 2017; 63(5): 1606-24.
[http://dx.doi.org/10.1287/mnsc.2016.2445]

[39] Liu X, Hu M, Helm JE, Lavieri MS, Skolarus TA. Missed opportunities in preventing hospital readmissions: Redesigning post-discharge checkup policies. Prod Oper Manag 2018; 27(12): 2226-50.
[http://dx.doi.org/10.1111/poms.12858]

[40] Kern LM, Bynum JP, Pincus HA. Care fragmentation, care continuity, and care coordination—how they differ and why it matters. JAMA internal medicine 2024 Mar 1; 184(3): 236-7.
[http://dx.doi.org/10.1001/jamainternmed.2023.7628]

[41] Bynum JP, Montoya A, Lawton EJ, Gibbons JB, Banerjee M, Meddings J, Norton EC. Accountable care organization attribution and post-acute skilled nursing facility outcomes for people living with dementia. J Ame Med Direct Assoc 2024 Jan 1; 25(1):53-7.
[http://dx.doi.org/10.1016/j.jamda.2023.10.031]

[42] Ciesielski TM, Henry TL, Fondahn ED. Accreditation and Health Policy and Their Impacts on Quality. Medical Clinics 2025 Sep 1; 109(5): 1103-16.
[http://dx.doi.org/10.1016/j.mcna.2025.02.009]

[43] Briggs ADM, Fraze TK, Glick AL, Beidler LB, Shortell SM, Fisher ES. How do accountable care organisations deliver preventive care services? A mixed-methods study. J Gen Intern Med 2019; 34(11): 2451-9.
[http://dx.doi.org/10.1007/s11606-019-05271-5] [PMID: 31432439]

[44] Fraze TK, Beidler LB, Briggs ADM, Colla CH. Translating evidence into practice: ACOs' use of care plans for patients with complex health needs. J Gen Intern Med 2021; 36(1): 147-53.
[http://dx.doi.org/10.1007/s11606-020-06122-4] [PMID: 33006083]

[45] Langenbrunner J, Cashin C, O'Dougherty S, Eds. Designing and implementing health care provider payment systems: how-to manuals. Washington (DC): World Bank Publications 2009.
[http://dx.doi.org/10.1596/978-0-8213-7815-1]

[46] Boachie MK, Amporfu E. Effect of capitation payment method on health outcomes, healthcare utilization, and referrals in Ghana. PLOS Global Public Health 2024; 4(6): e0002423.
[http://dx.doi.org/10.1371/journal.pgph.0002423] [PMID: 38905260]

[47] Gosden T, Forland F, Kristiansen I, *et al.* Capitation, salary, fee-for-service and mixed systems of payment: effects on the behaviour of primary care physicians. Cochrane Database Syst Rev 2000; 2000(3): CD002215.
[http://dx.doi.org/10.1002/14651858.CD002215] [PMID: 10908531]

[48] Wolfe PR, Moran DW. Global budgeting in the OECD countries. Health Care Financ Rev 1993; 14(3): 55-76.
[PMID: 10130584]

[49] Menifield C, Ed. Comparative public budgeting: a global perspective. Burlington (MA): Jones & Bartlett Publishers 2011.

[50] World Health Organization. Global patient safety action plan 2021-2030: towards eliminating avoidable harm in health care. World Health Organization; 2021 Aug 3.

[51] Britnell M. Human: solving the global workforce crisis in healthcare. Oxford University Press 2019.
[http://dx.doi.org/10.1093/oso/9780198836520.001.0001]

[52] Taylor LJ III. A comparison of capital budgeting models: local versus global viewpoints. Bus Process Manag J 1998; 4(4): 306-21.
[http://dx.doi.org/10.1108/14637159810238200]

[53] Ho A, De Jong M, Zhao Z, Eds. Performance budgeting reform: Theories and international practices. New York: Routledge 2019.
[http://dx.doi.org/10.4324/9781351055307]

[54] Dietz WH, Solomon LS, Pronk N, *et al.* An integrated framework for the prevention and treatment of obesity and its related chronic diseases. Health Aff (Millwood) 2015; 34(9): 1456-63.

[http://dx.doi.org/10.1377/hlthaff.2015.0371] [PMID: 26355046]

[55]   VanEpps EM, Troxel AB, Villamil E, *et al.* Financial incentives for chronic disease management: results and limitations of 2 randomised clinical trials with New York Medicaid patients. Am J Health Promot 2018; 32(7): 1537-43.
[http://dx.doi.org/10.1177/0890117117753986] [PMID: 29390862]

[56]   Abedalrhman K, Alzaydi A. Integration of fintech applications in public health strategies for sustainable development. SSRN 4970995.2024;
[http://dx.doi.org/10.2139/ssrn.4970995]

[57]   Wijaya LI, Zunairoh Z, Rianawati A, Prasetyo VR, Harianto I. Does financial technology matter? Evidence from the Indonesia healthcare industry during the COVID-19 pandemic. Sci Pap Univ Pardubice Ser D Fac Econ Adm 2022; 30(1): 1509.
[http://dx.doi.org/10.46585/sp30011509]

[58]   Guess GM, LeLoup LT. Comparative public budgeting: global perspectives on taxing and spending. Albany (NY): State University of New York Press 2010.

[59]   Nylen WR. Participatory Budgeting in Global Perspective. By Brian Wampler, Stephanie McNulty, and Michael Touchton. New York: Oxford University Press, 2021. 256p. $85.00 cloth. Perspect Polit 2022; 20(2): 747-8.
[http://dx.doi.org/10.1017/S1537592722000871]

[60]   Rane N, Choudhary S, Rane J. Blockchain and Artificial Intelligence (AI) integration for revolutionising security and transparency in finance. SSRN 4644253.2023;

[61]   Kokogho E, , Onwuzulike OC, Omowole BM, Ewim CP, Adeyanju MO. Blockchain technology and real-time auditing: Transforming financial transparency and fraud detection in the Fintech industry. Gulf J Adv Bus Res 2025; 3(2): 348-79.
[http://dx.doi.org/10.51594/gjabr.v3i2.88]

[62]   Cortez N. Patients without borders: the emerging global patient market and the evolution of modern health care. Ind Law J 2008; 83: 71.

[63]   Lo AW, Chaudhuri SE. Healthcare Finance: Modern Financial Analysis for Accelerating Biomedical Innovation. Princeton University Press; 2022 Nov 15.

[64]   Burtch G, Chan J. Investigating the relationship between medical crowdfunding and personal bankruptcy in the United States. Manage Inf Syst Q 2019; 43(1): 237-62.
[http://dx.doi.org/10.25300/MISQ/2019/14569]

[65]   Snyder J. Crowdfunding for medical care: ethical issues in an emerging health care funding practice. Hastings Cent Rep 2016; 46(6): 36-42.
[http://dx.doi.org/10.1002/hast.645] [PMID: 27875643]

[66]   Eling M, Nuessle D, Staubli J. The impact of artificial intelligence along the insurance value chain and on the insurability of risks. Geneva Pap Risk Insur Issues Pract 2022; 47(2): 205-41.
[http://dx.doi.org/10.1057/s41288-020-00201-7]

[67]   Kewal T, Saxena C. Digital disruption in insurance value chain. In: Proceedings of the International Conference on Innovative Computing and Communication (ICICC); 2024. Singapore: Springer 2024; pp. 173-185.

[68]   Tanwar T, Kumar UD, Mustafee N. Optimal package pricing in healthcare services. J Oper Res Soc 2020; 71(11): 1860-72.
[http://dx.doi.org/10.1080/01605682.2019.1654416]

[69]   Haggerty E. Healthcare and digital transformation. Netw Secur 2017; 2017(8): 7-11.
[http://dx.doi.org/10.1016/S1353-4858(17)30081-8]

[70]   Bhat JR, AlQahtani SA, Nekovee M. FinTech enablers, use cases, and role of future internet of things. J King Saud Univ Comput Inf Sci 2023; 35(1): 87-101.

[http://dx.doi.org/10.1016/j.jksuci.2022.08.033]

[71]   Ahmed MN, Anand A, Hussain MR, Ahmed MM, Khan IM, Rasool MA. Artificial intelligence in fintech: emerging trends and use cases. In: Proceedings of the 2024 IEEE 7th International Conference on Advanced Technologies, Signal and Image Processing (ATSIP); 2024 Jul 11; Sfax, Tunisia. Piscataway (NJ): IEEE 2024; pp. 459–464.

[72]   Hossain S, Ahmed A, Khadka U, Sarkar S, Khan N. AI-driven predictive analytics, healthcare outcomes, cost reduction, machine learning, patient monitoring. Adv Int J Multidis Res 2024; 2(5): 1-20.

[73]   Garg PP, Jayashree J, Vijayashree J. Revolutionizing healthcare: The transformative role of artificial intelligence. In: Responsible and Explainable Artificial Intelligence in Healthcare. Academic Press. 2025; pp. 1-23.
[http://dx.doi.org/10.1016/B978-0-443-24788-0.00001-7]

[74]   Gleißner W, Günther T, Walkshäusl C. Financial sustainability: measurement and empirical evidence. J Bus Econ 2022; 92(3): 467-516.
[http://dx.doi.org/10.1007/s11573-022-01081-0]

[75]   Agrawal R, Agrawal S, Samadhiya A, Kumar A, Luthra S, Jain V. Adoption of green finance and green innovation for achieving circularity: An exploratory review and future directions. Geoscience Frontiers 2024; 15(4): 101669.
[http://dx.doi.org/10.1016/j.gsf.2023.101669]

[76]   Zid C, Kasim N, Soomro AR. Effective project management approach to attain project success, based on cost-time-quality. Int J Project Organ Manage 2020; 12(2): 149-63.
[http://dx.doi.org/10.1504/IJPOM.2020.106376]

[77]   Obi LI, Arif M, Awuzie B, Islam R, Gupta AD, Walton R. Critical success factors for cost management in public-housing projects. Constr Innov 2021; 21(4): 625-47.
[http://dx.doi.org/10.1108/CI-10-2020-0166]

[78]   Oliveira MD, Bevan G. Modelling hospital costs to produce evidence for policies that promote equity and efficiency. Eur J Oper Res 2008; 185(3): 933-47.
[http://dx.doi.org/10.1016/j.ejor.2006.02.053]

[79]   Bacia JA. Developing effective budgeting and forecasting techniques. Res Invent J Curr Res Humanit Soc Sci 2024; 3(1): 71–5.

[80]   Wildavsky AB. Budgeting: a comparative theory of the budgeting process. New Brunswick (NJ): Transaction Publishers. 1986.

[81]   Zsidisin GA, Panelli A, Upton R. Purchasing organization involvement in risk assessments, contingency plans, and risk management: an exploratory study. Supply Chain Manag 2000; 5(4): 187-98.
[http://dx.doi.org/10.1108/13598540010347307]

[82]   Firoozi AA, Firoozi AA. Risk management and contingency planning. In: Revolutionizing civil engineering with neuromorphic computing. Cham: Springer 2024; pp. 73-80.
[http://dx.doi.org/10.1007/978-3-031-71097-1_9]

[83]   Gautam A, Khan ZA, Gani A, Asjad M. Identification, ranking and prioritization of Key Performance Indicators for evaluating greenness of manufactured products. Green Techno Sus 2025; 3(1): 100114.
[http://dx.doi.org/10.1016/j.grets.2024.100114]

[84]   Hristov I, Chirico A. The role of sustainability key performance indicators (KPIs) in implementing sustainable strategies. Sustainability (Basel) 2019; 11(20): 5742.
[http://dx.doi.org/10.3390/su11205742]

[85]   Marrucci L, Daddi T, Iraldo F. Creating environmental performance indicators to assess corporate sustainability and reward employees. Ecol Indic 2024; 158: 111489.
[http://dx.doi.org/10.1016/j.ecolind.2023.111489]

[86] Ryszawska B. Sustainability transition needs sustainable finance. Coper J Fin Acc 2016; 5(1): 185-94. [http://dx.doi.org/10.12775/CJFA.2016.011]

[87] Passoja P. Budgeting and forecasting application development: an evaluation. Master's thesis. Tampere (Finland): Tampere University of Applied Sciences 2015.

[88] Ursu C. Navigating the journey in budgeting: major steps in making a complex subject manageable. 1st ed. Lanham (MD): Rowman & Littlefield Publishers; 2023 May 8.

[89] Nazara DS, Oktoriza LA, Rahimah R. Navigating the financial landscape: the importance of budgeting. J Eco Bus Acc (costing) 2024; 7(4): 8245-9. [https://doi.org/10.31539/costing.v7i4.10582]

[90] Stobierski T. Financial performance measures managers should monitor. Harvard Business School. 2020 May 5.

[91] Mtau TT, Rahul NA. Optimizing business performance through KPI alignment: a comprehensive analysis of key performance indicators and strategic objectives. Amer J Indus Bus Manag 2024; 14(1): 66-82.
[http://dx.doi.org/10.4236/ajibm.2024.141003]

[92] Kusek JZ, Rist RC. Ten steps to a results-based monitoring and evaluation system: a handbook for development practitioners. World Bank Publications; 2004 Jun 15.

[93] Clements P. Book review: a handbook for development practitioners: ten steps to a results-based monitoring and evaluation system. Am J Eval 2005; 26(2): 278-80.
[http://dx.doi.org/10.1177/1098214005276282]

[94] Lindner L, Lorenzoni L. Innovative providers' payment models for promoting value-based health systems: start small, prove value, and scale up. OECD Health Working Papers 2023; 154. Paris: OECD Publishing. [http://dx.doi.org/10.1787/627fe490-en]

[95] van Elten HJ, Howard SW, De Loo I, Schaepkens F. Reflections on managing the performance of value-based healthcare: a scoping review. Int J Health Policy Manag 2023; 12: 7366.
[http://dx.doi.org/10.34172/ijhpm.2023.7366] [PMID: 37579381]

[96] Cossio-Gil Y, Omara M, Watson C, *et al.* The roadmap for implementing value-based healthcare in European university hospitals—consensus report and recommendations. Value Health 2022; 25(7): 1148-56.
[http://dx.doi.org/10.1016/j.jval.2021.11.1355] [PMID: 35779941]

[97] Anawade PA, Sharma D, Gahane S. A comprehensive review on exploring the impact of telemedicine on healthcare accessibility. Cureus 2024; 16(3): e55996.
[http://dx.doi.org/10.7759/cureus.55996] [PMID: 38618307]

[98] Al-Saleem AI, Aldakheel MK. Barriers to workforce-driven innovation in healthcare. Cureus 2024; 16(10): e72316.
[PMID: 39450215]

[99] Khalili H. Transforming health care delivery: innovations in payment models for interprofessional team-based care. N C Med J 2024; 85(3): 173-7.
[http://dx.doi.org/10.18043/001c.117089] [PMID: 39437346]

[100] Das S, Dey A, Pal A, Roy N. Applications of artificial intelligence in machine learning: review and prospect. Int J Comput Appl 2015; 115(9): 31-41.
[http://dx.doi.org/10.5120/20182-2402]

[101] Ullah Z, Al-Turjman F, Mostarda L, Gagliardi R. Applications of Artificial Intelligence and Machine learning in smart cities. Comput Commun 2020; 154: 313-23.
[http://dx.doi.org/10.1016/j.comcom.2020.02.069]

[102] Iqbal MJ, Javed Z, Sadia H, *et al.* Clinical applications of artificial intelligence and machine learning in cancer diagnosis: looking into the future. Cancer Cell Int 2021; 21(1): 270.
[http://dx.doi.org/10.1186/s12935-021-01981-1] [PMID: 34020642]

CHAPTER 7

Training Healthcare Professionals in Technology Adoption

Shaweta Sharma[1], Akhil Sharma[2], Ashish Verma[3], Akanksha Sharma[2] and Rakesh Patel[4,*]

[1] *School of Medical and Allied Sciences, Galgotias University, Yamuna Expressway, Gautam Buddha Nagar, Uttar Pradesh 201310, India*

[2] *R.J. College of Pharmacy, Raipur, Gharbara, Tappal, Khair, Uttar Pradesh 202165, India*

[3] *Mangalmay Pharmacy College, Greater Noida, Uttar Pradesh 201306, India*

[4] *Malwa Institute of Pharmaceutical Science, Indore, Madhya Pradesh 452001, India*

Abstract: Technology has made advancements in healthcare that focus more on service delivery and giving patients efficient, high-access services. Technological advancements have significantly changed the way services are provided in the healthcare sector, making it more efficient and accessible while ultimately improving patient outcomes. However, these improvements must be accompanied by training programs for healthcare providers to learn how to use new technologies. This chapter will provide insight into the significant importance of training as a means through which healthcare providers can be empowered to maximise technology in care delivery. It offers key insights into some of the most critical healthcare technologies, such as electronic health records (EHR), telemedicine, artificial intelligence (AI), wearable devices, and blockchain, highlighting their ability to reduce workflows and improve decision-making. Healthcare professionals face several challenges in getting on board with technology, which this chapter touches upon, including resistance to change, lack of technical skills, integration barriers, and resource constraints. A needs assessment approach is also offered, focusing on tailoring training to the specific needs and context of different roles across healthcare teams. Strategies like hands-on workshops, simulation-based learning, and AI-powered adaptive training are proposed to enable effective knowledge transfer and practical competency development. The chapter highlights successful technology training program implementations in various healthcare settings through case studies and best practices. The discussion highlights how training can lead to better care, fewer mistakes, and caring satisfaction. AI advancements can drive personalised learning experiences, broaden training access in underserved areas, and encourage cross-sector policies for sustained education. It offers a significant perspective on how structured training is essential in preparing healthcare

* **Corresponding author Rakesh Patel:** Malwa Institute of Pharmaceutical Science, Indore, Madhya Pradesh 452001, India; E-mail: patelcip@gmail.com

Akhil Sharma, Shaweta Sharma, Pankaj Kumar Singh & Neeraj Kumar Fuloria (Eds.)

professionals to adapt to and flourish in an increasingly technology-driven environment.

Keywords: Accessibility, Efficiency, Healthcare, Innovation, Optimised healthcare systems, Sigital health transformation, Technology adoption.

INTRODUCTION

In healthcare, digital adoption transforms existing care processes to make them more effective and efficient by incorporating new technologies. These new tools and platforms allow healthcare organisations to conduct more transactional administrative activities, *e.g.*, scheduling additional appointments virtually, responding more rapidly to patient questions, better managing staff availability, and diversifying routes for treatments and payments [1].

The notable emergence of new healthcare applications and services enables healthcare organisations to create new partnerships, be proactive, and reimagine care and communication with patients. A digital adoption strategy will help ensure that healthcare workers and patients are up to speed with these new technology developments and ready for a shift without disruptions [2].

Training healthcare professionals is essential for improving the effectiveness and quality of health services, continuing education opportunities, but also hands-on experience to provide practical exposure and real-world assessments of patient outcomes. With continuous professional development, the workforce is prepared to use telemedicine, artificial intelligence, and precision medicine [3, 4]. Theoretical learning and practical training develop the critical thinking and problem-solving skills that underpin patient care. Furthermore, interprofessional training facilitates teamwork and communication, which helps strengthen cooperation in care. Soft skills training on empathy, cultural competence and patient education is emphasised to promote holistic care delivery by addressing diverse patient needs that foster trust and satisfaction [5, 6].

Benefits of Digital Adoption in Healthcare

The healthcare field has historically been slow to adopt new technology compared with other industries. This is partly due to its highly regulated nature and a patchwork of legacy systems that lack data interoperability.

Yet the pandemic left these organisations with no choice but to adopt a quick and consumer-market-enabled service approach (which prioritises increased transparency, availability, and accessibility). Moreover, burnout among healthcare personnel increased the need for enhanced resources and tools to avoid staff shortages, improve processes, and reduce financial strain on the sector [7, 8]. The benefits of digital adoption in healthcare are summarised in Fig. (**1**).

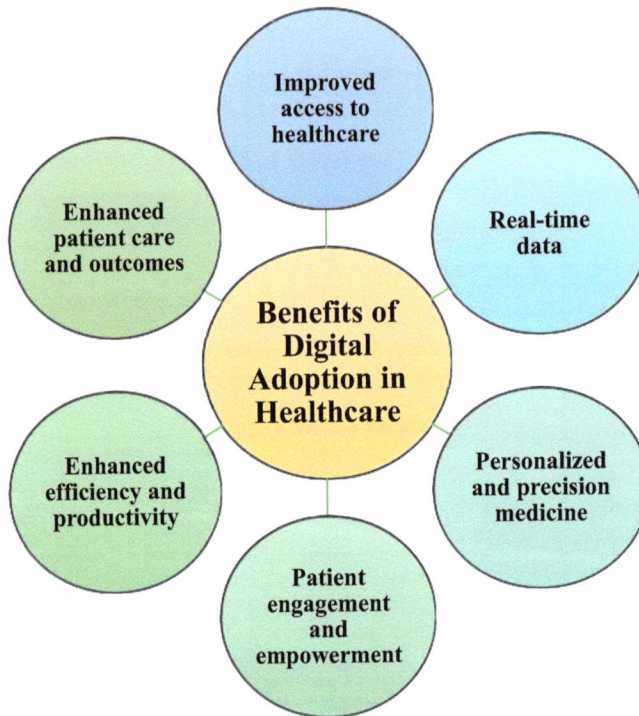

Fig. (1). Benefits of digital adoption in healthcare.

Digital adoption allows the healthcare industry to be agile and forward-thinking, giving organisations the following benefits:

Enhanced Patient Care and Outcomes

Patient care is fast transitioning to digital channels that provide easy ways to monitor health, schedule appointments, and receive treatments. Wearable healthcare devices such as smartwatches and biosensors capture data on a patient's mobility patterns, heart rate, and temperature so that patients with chronic medical conditions can be monitored remotely [9].

This innovation enables healthcare staff to reduce the manual administrative tasks required while giving patients greater flexibility in receiving timely treatment or consultation *via* virtual meetings, even if they cannot attend an on-site appointment [10].

Improved Access to Healthcare

Digitised healthcare processes make delaying treatment harder because of location, scheduling conflicts, or a limited price range for different treatment methods, and the healthcare professionals' supply.

However, digital interoperability in the healthcare space has been on the rise, enabling healthcare startups to introduce new solutions quickly that increase access to healthcare [11].

Real-time Data

Digital adoption enables healthcare providers to extract more excellent value from patient data. Paper-based processes and manual data management have historically diverted hospital staff from providing quality care, decreasing overall efficiency [12].

Legacy healthcare solutions such as legacy hospital information systems, electronic health record systems, revenue cycle management software, and the like are often seen as separate applications. Moreover, no healthcare organisation can conduct a scaled analysis from multiple data points without integrations between different software solutions.

Conversely, the healthcare technology ecosystem today promotes easy interaction. By training employees and patients to leverage these technologies, hospitals can automate data collection, make quicker decisions, and provide real-time information [13, 14].

Personalised and Precision Medicine

Healthcare providers have access to a wealth of molecular-genetic data that informs treatment plans based on a biological characteristic a patient may possess.

This medicine still has a long way to go in terms of accessibility. Streamlining healthcare data across multiple systems and devices makes the implementation of more robust digital management processes and regulatory frameworks essential. The use of digital tools to collect, store, and interpret unstandardised data safely creates more options for patients to take ownership of their data and collaborate better with their healthcare teams [15, 16].

Enhanced Efficiency and Productivity

Healthcare organisations use technology to streamline operational processes, eliminate manual administrative tasks, and fill digital literacy gaps [17].

Patient Engagement and Empowerment

Consumer-centric health technologies provide a significant boost to patient access to data and services anywhere, propelling consumer-driven healthcare. Startup companies such as Hims & Hers were formed to encourage consumers to be more involved in their healthcare decisions *via* telemedicine [18].

Role of Healthcare Professionals in Technology Adoption

Healthcare professionals must adopt the technology and integrate it into their everyday lives. Their willingness to embrace innovation guarantees the successful implementation of advanced tools like electronic health records (EHRs), telemedicine platforms, and AI-driven diagnostic systems. Serving as primary users, clinicians contribute to the design and function of technology by guiding its clinical relevance and fit with existing workflow demands [19, 20].

Their role in educating patients about new technologies builds trust and encourages patient engagement in digital health initiatives. Furthermore, professionals drive the change of technology by having their part to play in training, disseminating best practices, and resolving resistance issues in their organisations. Healthcare professionals are grooved at the intersection of innovation and practicality, and by encouraging technology adoption, they facilitate the transfer between the two to enhance patient care and system efficiency, ultimately [21, 22].

Healthcare systems are being built and reformed with modern aspirations of efficiency, accessibility, and optimised delivery to address the expanding needs of diverse populations. Efficiency incorporates process automation with technology, eliminating duplicate work and improving resource distribution so healthcare practitioners can spend more time caring for patients [23].

Accessibility ensures that individuals, regardless of location or socio-economic status, can access quality healthcare through mobile clinics, telemedicine and community health programs. Optimised delivery enables timely and accurate treatments by focusing on patient-centred care through data analytics, personalised medicine and evidence-based practices. Achieving these goals will result in fair healthcare systems where the focus on outcomes, costs and broader satisfaction is balanced [24, 25]. The role of healthcare professionals in the adoption of technology is summarised in Table **1**.

Table 1. Role of healthcare professionals in the adoption of technology [26 - 33].

Healthcare Professional	Role in Technology Adoption
Clinicians (Doctors)	• Lead the implementation of novel technologies into clinical settings. • Offer feedback on the usability and effectiveness of the technology. • Adopt technology that facilitates clinical decision-making and patient care.
Nurses	• Serve as frontline users of various healthcare technologies (*e.g.*, patient monitoring, electronic health records). • Provide support for patient training in digital health tools (*e.g.*, telehealth). • Track technology usage and give feedback for improvement.
Healthcare Administrators	• Manage the integration and use of health technologies (*e.g.*, EHR systems, telemedicine platforms). • Organize staff training programs to ensure compliance with regulations. • Manage resources for technology infrastructure and support.
IT and Support Staff	• Ensure the infrastructure of healthcare technology systems (*e.g.*, EHR, telemedicine). • Ensure technical support and troubleshooting for health technology users. • Handle data security and privacy protocols to keep patient information safe.
Medical Technologists	• Employ sophisticated diagnostic technologies (*e.g.*, imaging systems, laboratory software). • Ensure accurate and efficient use of technological tools for testing and diagnostics.
Pharmacists	• Embed medication management technologies, like computerised prescription systems. • Ensure patients benefit from technology-assisted drug therapies and counselling.
Educators and Trainers	• Develop and deliver training programs for healthcare professionals on new technologies. • Support adopting new tools through hands-on workshops and ongoing education.

TECHNOLOGY USED IN HEALTHCARE

Technology integration in healthcare has revolutionised how services are delivered, enhancing efficiency, accuracy, and patient outcomes. Technological innovations used in healthcare are described below and depicted in Fig. (**2**).

Digital Health Tools

Electronic Health Records (EHR) revolutionised the health sector by consolidating patient data electronically, giving healthcare providers easy access to a vast spectrum of patient medical histories. This enhances coordination between medical teams and reduces duplication and errors in diagnosis and treatment. Likewise, mobile health applications enable patients with tools to track fitness, manage chronic conditions, and receive personalised health advice. Moreover, these apps provide a better channel for communication between patients and providers, promoting a collaborative approach to health management [34, 35].

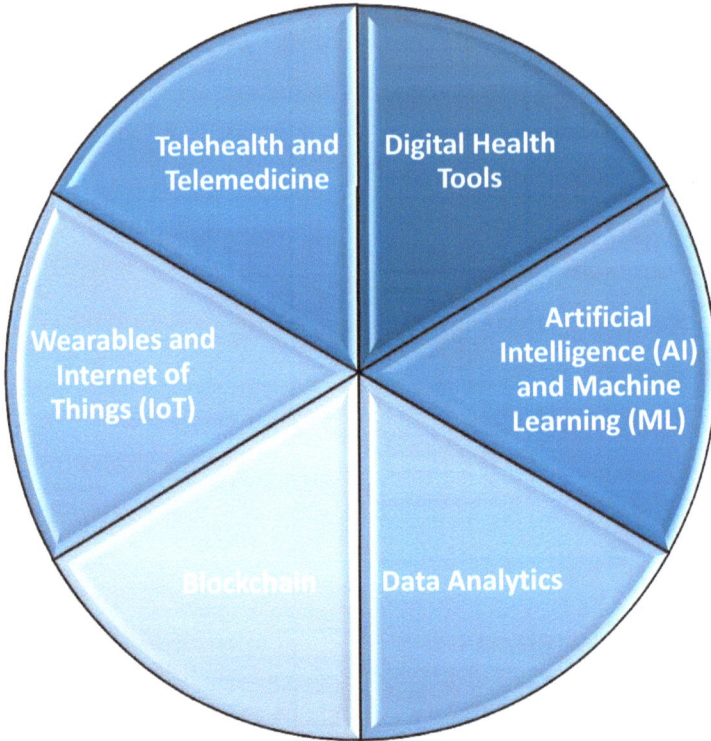

Fig. (2). Technology used in healthcare.

Telehealth and Telemedicine

Patients and healthcare providers have connected through virtual consultations, giving a massive advantage to those living in remote or underserved areas. Telehealth helps to avoid unnecessary resources and time by reducing the need for a physical visit and improving care delivery. Remote patient monitoring builds on this by using devices that continuously monitor vital health information such as blood pressure and glucose levels. This was particularly so in the case of chronic diseases, where timely medical intervention can ensure better patient outcomes [36, 37].

Artificial Intelligence (AI) and Machine Learning (ML)

AI and ML have become vital in increasing the precision of healthcare. AI systems leverage massive datasets in clinical settings to suggest evidence-based treatment options and identify possible health risks. ML diagnostics and treatment planning algorithms detect patterns from medical imaging, genomic data, and laboratory results, enabling earlier and more accurate diagnoses. These factors directly contribute to personalised treatment plans that can be much more effective [38, 39].

Wearables and the Internet of Things (IoT)

Wearables are smart devices like watches and fitness trackers that monitor live data such as heart rate, sleep activity, and physical exercise. These data may indicate an early risk of poor health and allow for better intervention. Additionally, devices powered by IoT help drive patient engagement by motivating patients to be physically involved in tracking their health and following treatment plans, thus creating a feeling that they control their well-being [40, 41].

Blockchain

Blockchain represents solutions to significant pain points in healthcare, especially around data security and transparency. In contrast, its decentralised system encrypts sensitive patient data for robust protection and minimises the risk of a breach. Moreover, due to its tamper-proof nature for transactions, blockchain enables a transparent billing process that minimises cases of fraud and ensures clarity of healthcare payments made [42, 43].

Data Analytics

Predictive analytics uses historical and real-time data to identify trends in the health of populations, predict which ones are at risk, and target preventive care initiatives. This improves decision-making for providers and policymakers alike. By harnessing insights from aggregate data, population health management enables the creation of new healthcare interventions, addresses public health challenges, and focuses on resource allocation for improved outcomes at the community level. Together, they improve efficiency, accuracy and accessibility by tackling different facets of healthcare, leading to significant changes in patient care [44, 45].

CHALLENGES IN TECHNOLOGY ADOPTION

Healthcare technology adoption challenges must be overcome to facilitate successful healthcare technology integration. One major challenge faced by health teams is overcoming this resistance and getting professionals to update out-of-date practices for more innovative technologies, mainly since many have been used for years. This resistance is frequently rooted in unfamiliarity, anxiety over change or doubt about the advantages of new technologies. This must be overcome with thoughtful change management strategies and continual training [46].

The other challenge is that the healthcare staff often lacks technical skills, including those who are not trained to operate various electronic health data and AI tools. These technologies can not reach their full potential without working on training them properly. Moreover, integrating these with existing systems is often challenging. Legacy healthcare systems are often not compatible with new technology, which can create inefficiencies, data silos, or disrupt workflows. These gaps need to be bridged by interoperable solutions that enable smooth transitions [47].

Another obstacle to the adoption of technology in healthcare is the financial aspect. The investment required for implementation and maintenance can be excessively high, especially in smaller practices or resource-limited environments. Affordable, scalable solutions are critical to addressing this challenge. Finally, data privacy and security are always concerns in digital healthcare [48].

As patient information becomes more digitised, the risk of cyberattacks and data breaches increases, highlighting the importance of implementing secure cybersecurity measures, encryption protocols, and compliance standards to safeguard sensitive data and preserve patient trust. The appropriate solutions to these challenges lie in an ecosystem-wide response requiring stakeholders, investment in training, and secure, interoperable technologies [49, 50].

TRAINING NEEDS ASSESSMENT

Healthcare professionals, in particular, will need to undergo this training if emerging technology is to ensure better health outcomes for our communities. It includes a few basic steps to determine competencies, identify gaps, and close them through training so that you have the right employees for the job [51, 52].

Identifying Competency Gaps

The first step in a training needs assessment (TNA) is identifying competency gaps within the workforce. This requires assessing existing skills and comparing them to those needed for new technologies and changing healthcare approaches. It helps illuminate areas where healthcare professionals may not be as skilled, whether that's using digital tools, understanding new treatment protocols, or navigating data systems. Recognising these gaps enables organisations to focus training efforts and create targeted programs to fill these shortcomings [53, 54].

Role-Specific Requirements

Another essential element of the training needs assessment is a sensible approach to data generation, including identifying role-specific demands in healthcare contexts. When adopting new technology, the needs can vary according to the style employed in hospitals, such as doctors, nurses, technicians, or administrative staff. For example, physicians might need training on AI-based diagnostic tools, while administrative staff would require knowledge in managing electronic health records (EHRs) and telehealth platforms. Customising training according to these requirements equips both with the knowledge and support they need in their roles [55, 56].

Addressing Generational and Cultural Differences

Finally, it is essential to consider generational and cultural differences in the training process. Different generations of healthcare professionals may have varying levels of comfort and familiarity with technology. Older employees are generally more resistant to change and may even be intimidated by new digital tools, but younger employees are usually tech-savvy. Similarly, misalignments with one or more of the eight cultural differences could lead to mismatched learning styles and communication preferences. Providing flexible, culturally attuned and accessible training methodologies like task-based workshops, webinars, E-learning modules, or mentorship programs will promote an environment of inclusivity around learning that accommodates the workforce's diverse needs [57, 58].

TRAINING STRATEGIES AND TOOLS

Thus, effective training strategies and tools are critical to enabling healthcare professionals to embrace technology and modern processes and improve patient care. These strategies must address a variety of learning types and ensure that all have the opportunity to become well-prepared for their role in an increasingly technology-centric health system [59]. Training strategies and tools used in healthcare are summarised in Fig. (3).

Learning Approaches

Diverse learning methods can encourage practical experience and enable well-rounded learning. They provide practical exposure to new tools and systems, letting learners practice using technology in real-life scenarios. This method boosts retention and confidence in the use of new skills. Simulation-based training provides an environment for professionals to experience complex healthcare scenarios, like emergency procedures or surgery, without consequence [60, 61].

The simulations assist in improving decision-making and technical skills. Healthcare organisations have embraced technology to provide training in innovative ways, such as virtual reality simulations or e-learning modules that allow employees to learn at their own pace. Such platforms can be a great way to stay current concerning continuous professional development in a rapidly changing technological environment [62, 63].

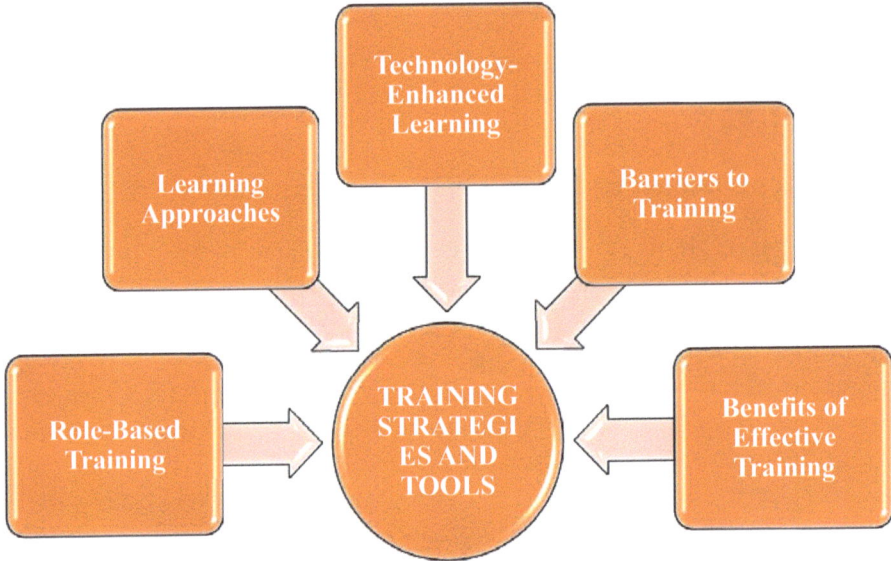

Fig. (3). Training strategies and tools.

Role-Based Training

Role-based training helps customise educational content for healthcare staff's unique needs and responsibilities. For clinicians, the focus might be on training related to advanced diagnostic tools, patient management software, and clinical decision support systems. Nurses will need training on mobile health applications, patient monitoring technologies, and telemedicine protocols. Administrators need training on managing electronic health records, complying with regulations, and overseeing telehealth platforms. IT and support personnel need to obtain technical knowledge about system integration, troubleshooting, cybersecurity, and data management. With the distinct needs of each profession in mind, organisations ensure that every individual is prepared to perform their duties efficiently and effectively [64 - 66].

Technology-Enhanced Learning

Technology-enhanced learning tools provide innovative ways to excite learners about learning, tempting them into the classroom with these familiar digital gadgets. Another excellent technology for training applications is VR (virtual reality) and AR (augmented reality). For example, VR can replicate intricate surgeries or emergencies so experts can practice without consequences, whereas AR can cover vital details. Gamification adds an element of engagement by turning learning into a game-like experience that makes skill acquisition more interactive and enjoyable, often resulting in enhanced retention. Finally, AI-enabled adaptive learning adjusts training pathways according to the progress and performance of the learner, thereby ensuring an individualised experience catered to unique needs, strengths, and shortcomings. When incorporated effectively into training programs, these strategies facilitate the smooth adoption of technology and help establish a culture of continuous improvement, keeping healthcare organisations agile and engaged [67 - 69].

Benefits of Effective Training

Good healthcare training has several benefits that directly affect both the professionals involved and the healthcare system itself. Some of the most significant advantages are improved efficiency in healthcare delivery and the adoption of specialist workers, who can be trained to use technology more effectively. The results are faster decision-making and better productivity [70].

A well-trained workforce also contributes directly to better patient care and safety, as staff will be better prepared and use advanced tools to develop best practices and respond to patients quickly and more effectively. Comprehensive training equips technologies with proficiency, thus reducing potential errors during usage. In addition, they are now adept at using digital systems, medical devices, and other technologies [71].

Finally, proper training increases job satisfaction and retention. Healthcare professionals who feel competent and supported are more likely to continue working in the field. This feeling of achievement contributes to better job satisfaction and retention, which benefits both staff and patients because they both thrive in an environment of constant development [72, 73].

Barriers to Training

Practical training is vital to enhance healthcare practices; however, several challenges hinder successful implementations. Financial and resource constraints are one of the key obstacles. Some healthcare organisations, especially those with limited budgets or in low-resource settings, may have difficulty investing in all the resources that comprehensive training programs require, including technology investment, staff time, and external expertise [74].

Additionally, organisational resistance can be a significant hurdle. Healthcare organisations or leadership teams may not want to invest in training because they do not know how valuable it will be, or are afraid of interrupting business as usual. This resistance can slow down or even wholly hinder the adoption of critical technological progress. Time constraints for healthcare staff represent another barrier. These healthcare professionals are already burdened with heavy workloads, making it challenging to allocate time for education. Consequently, it delays technology adoption and diminishes the overall impact of learning programs [75].

Finally, insufficient opportunities for ongoing skill-building can lead to stagnation in professional growth. Lifelong learning is vital when working in fast-moving domains such as healthcare technology. Even then, staff not only need structured programs, mentorship, or opportunities for ongoing education, but they also must keep pace with the latest tools, techniques, and best practices in software development so that their initial training investment continues to pay dividends. Breaking through these barriers needs planning, resource allocation, and a company culture emphasising continuous improvement and professional development [76, 77].

CASE STUDIES AND BEST PRACTICES

Examining case studies and best practices for implementing healthcare technology training provides valuable insights into practical strategies and successful outcomes.

Successful Implementations in Hospitals

For example, large hospitals have successfully implemented electronic health records (EHR) and telehealth. Already, institutions that adopted robust, role-specific programs to skill up their medical and administrative staff are enjoying the benefits of enhanced operational efficiency, improved patient care, and seamless transitions in operations toward digital workflows [78].

For instance, a U.S. hospital network that implements EHRs across its system offers in-depth training and simulation-based workshops for clinicians, nurses, and support staff. Consequently, the hospital saw a drastic decrease in data entry errors, enhanced department communication, and improved patient outcomes. This successful implementation highlighted the need for customisation-based training for each role and, more importantly, ongoing support [79].

Public-Private Collaborations for Training

Public-private partnerships can play a key role at scale to support training programs for healthcare professionals. In one instance, a public health department and a private technology company worked together to launch a national telemedicine training initiative in India. This program was designed to train health workers in rural areas on how to perform remote consultations. The private partner offered the technological backbone, while the public sector contributed logistical support and access to health care personnel. Through joint efforts and collaborations, the program significantly increased the availability of telemedicine tools serving rural communities across several states while providing assistance with digital skill development for healthcare professionals working in low-resource environments [80, 81].

Innovations in Low-Resource Settings

Innovative training models have emerged in low-resource settings, where traditional training methods may not be feasible due to financial constraints or limited infrastructure. In Africa, for example, a mobile-based training program was developed to help healthcare workers learn how to use medical devices and digital health tools. They could access training materials, videos and interactive quizzes *via* mobile phones. This method offered an inexpensive, scalable approach to training in rural areas. Community health workers (CHWs) to provide peer-based training on mobile health applications and diagnostic tools are also confirmed as a success story. This method utilised local expertise and networks, which increased both the accessibility and cultural relevance of the training [82, 83].

Case Studies Related to Several Diseases

Effective management of both communicable and non-communicable diseases, such as tuberculosis, cholera, AIDS, cancer, arthritis, blindness, and renal failure, requires the training of healthcare professionals (HCPs) in technology adoption. This summary features a series of case studies and reflections on how the training initiatives have adapted for each disease area [84].

Tuberculosis (TB)

The World Health Organization (WHO) prepares the taxonomy for incorporating digital technologies into TB programs. Mobile health applications, such as SMS reminders and digital monitoring systems, can play a crucial role in improving communication between patients and healthcare providers. An Ethiopian study noted that HCPs were highly willing to use mobile-based SMS technology with determinants like effort expectancy and facilitating conditions, which substantially affected their intention to adopt these instruments. A systematic review showed that training HCPs and volunteers resulted in significantly higher TB case detection rates, underscoring the utility of educational interventions to manage healthcare results better [85, 86].

Cholera

Although no specific case studies on cholera were featured in the search results, applicable general principles from other disease areas can be extrapolated. Incorporating rapid response and effective communication technologies into training programs can help manage cholera outbreaks, as mobile health solutions provide another avenue for real-time data collection and dissemination during epidemics [87].

AIDS

Many training initiatives for AIDS management adopt digital health strategies analogous to those for TB. Telehealth-based programs have become prominent, especially during the COVID-19 pandemic, which requires remote patient monitoring and virtual visits. Such a transition at the time prepared HCPs to adapt and embrace new technologies, highlighting the need for structured training programs covering the basics of telehealth and patient engagement strategies [88].

Cancer

In oncology, the implementation of technology is becoming more critical for telehealth and remote monitoring of patients. Developing training programs to facilitate the oncologists' proficient utilisation of electronic health records (EHRs) and telehealth platforms. Integrating digital tools into oncological treatment pathways can improve patient outcomes through enhanced communication, education and adherence [89].

Arthritis

Training HCPs in wearable technology and mobile applications can help improve patient self-management for chronic diseases like arthritis. Educational programs can focus on interpreting data from these devices and personalising treatment plans appropriately [90].

Blindness

In ophthalmology, integrating technology into training programs (*e.g.*, teleophthalmology) improves access to care for patients with visual impairments.

Healthcare professionals are trained to use digital imaging tools and remote consultation systems to diagnose and manage eye diseases [91].

Kidney Failure

Kidney failure is often treated with complex treatment regimens that need to be monitored frequently. Training HCPs in telehealth technologies can help manage patients' conditions through remote consultations and monitoring systems alerting the provider to changes in a patient's critical health status [92].

Utilising technology in healthcare is essential for better managing various diseases. Disease area-specific case studies demonstrate the effectiveness of structured training programs to facilitate the appropriate use of digital tools among healthcare professionals. With healthcare working towards a greater alignment of digital solutions, continued education will be key to preparing HCPs for the demands of both communicable and non-communicable diseases [93, 94].

FUTURE DIRECTIONS

As technology advances and healthcare needs change, the future of training for healthcare professionals is changing. To move healthcare forward toward these and other new technologies, a few main areas will guide training programs to enable healthcare professionals to be prepared for the challenges ahead [95].

The sustainability and effectiveness of training initiatives require the formulation of sensible policies supporting healthcare training. Furthermore, policymakers and regulators must create an environment encouraging continuous learning and skills development among healthcare staff. Such policies might include funding training programmes, accreditation of educational institutes, and standardised certifications to ensure maintaining competency levels in the workforce [96].

Also, policymakers need to find ways to overcome technology access issues so that all healthcare professionals share the bandwidth and smartphones required to use the new tools and systems. By providing supportive frameworks, policymakers can encourage a culture of lifelong learning in healthcare [97].

Another exciting frontier for healthcare training is the integration of AI and automation into personalised learning. For the learner, AI-powered platforms can provide personalised learning opportunities by adjusting according to the learner's pace, preferences and progress. Using intelligent algorithms, these systems can pinpoint student knowledge gaps, recommend relevant learning materials, and provide personalised feedback [98].

AI can also be used, for instance, to integrate and intelligently design training modules that accommodate the clinician's previous knowledge and skills so that they learn more efficiently and quickly adopt complex technologies. This type of managed learning will ensure medical staff are well-versed with the latest treatment trends and best practices, raising industry quality [99].

Further training programs in rural and underserved communities are needed. Communities like these often have little access to educational resources, fewer healthcare professionals, and poor infrastructure. To solve these problems, health technologies, telemedicine, and remote learning platforms must be leveraged to reach healthcare workers in these areas [100].

Virtual workshops, webinars, and mobile apps can deliver critical training without requiring employees to travel long distances. This gap can be further closed through public-private partnerships, which help provide the necessary infrastructure and expertise to scale high-quality, accessible training right at the doorstep of underserved communities [101].

Ongoing advances in training methodologies will also be necessary to prepare healthcare professionals for the new and emerging challenges they will face. Given the rapid pace of technological development, training programs in innovation must be dynamic and flexible. In the future, blended learning modalities will be implemented with a combination of in-person and online education, coupled with virtual simulations applied to the training approach [102].

Simulation-based training, VR, and AR will become more commonplace, offering immersive and interactive learning experiences. Additionally, data analytics will help track learning outcomes and identify areas for improvement, ensuring that training programs are continually refined to meet the evolving needs of healthcare systems [103].

CONCLUSION

Successful technology implementation in health care mostly depends on the training and empowerment of health practitioners. This remote training will help ensure that healthcare workers have the digital skills necessary to make innovation a practical reality (and safeguard against potential misuse). Tropes of structured training programs, interdisciplinary collaboration, and the need for continuous learning have been emphasised in this chapter to cultivate a culture of technological proficiency and adaptability. These advancements make it easier for healthcare professionals to work efficiently, leading to better patient outcomes when paired with the right tools for quality care. Nevertheless, this is only possible by overcoming the barriers that prevent it, resistance to change, limited use of resources and differences in the level of digital literacy among professionals. Such challenges can be addressed through targeted strategies like experiential learning, mentorship programs, innovative educational tools, and virtual simulations. Future healthcare systems will be more tech-centric, but we must ensure that technology enables actual patient-centric care rather than distracting from it. As healthcare organisations stand to benefit immensely from the potential that technology offers, human resources should be carefully and thoughtfully managed so managers can ensure a well-trained, agile, and tech-savvy workforce. In the future, continued investment in the training and development of healthcare professionals will be the cornerstone for harnessing technology to provide adequate healthcare.

CONSENT FOR PUBLICATON

All authors have given their consent for publication. The authors authorised Rakesh Patel to handle all correspondences.

ACKNOWLEDGEMENTS

Authors are highly thankful to their Universities/Colleges for providing library facilities for the literature survey.

REFERENCES

[1] Marcos-Pablos S, Juanes-Mendez JA, Eds. Technological Adoption and Trends in Health Sciences Teaching, Learning, and Practice. IGI Global 2022.
[http://dx.doi.org/10.4018/978-1-7998-8871-0]

[2] Rangarajan A. Emerging trends in healthcare adoption of wireless body area networks. Biomed Instrum Technol 2016; 50(4): 264-76.
[http://dx.doi.org/10.2345/0899-8205-50.4.264] [PMID: 27413830]

[3] Niazi AS. Training and development strategy and its role in organisational performance. J Pub Admin Gover 2011; 1(2): 42.

[4] Mayo A. Creating a training and development strategy. Hyderabad: Universities Press; 1998. 1998.

[5] Utley J, Mathena C, Gunaldo T, Eds. Interprofessional education and collaboration: an evidence-based approach to optimising health care. Champaign (IL): Human Kinetics; 2020. 2020.

[6] Chang E, Simon M, Dong X. Integrating cultural humility into health care professional education and training. Adv Health Sci Educ Theory Pract 2012; 17(2): 269-78.
[http://dx.doi.org/10.1007/s10459-010-9264-1] [PMID: 21161680]

[7] Imison C, Castle-Clarke S, Watson R, Edwards N. Delivering the benefits of digital health care. London: Nuffield Trust; 2016 Feb.

[8] Landers M, Dorsey R, Saria S. Digital endpoints: definition, benefits, and current barriers in accelerating development and adoption. Digit Biomark 2021; 5(3): 216-23.
[http://dx.doi.org/10.1159/000517885] [PMID: 34703976]

[9] Hilty DM, Armstrong CM, Edwards-Stewart A, Gentry MT, Luxton DD, Krupinski EA. Sensor, wearable, and remote patient monitoring competencies for clinical care and training: scoping review. J Technol Behav Sci 2021; 6(2): 252-77.

[http://dx.doi.org/10.1007/s41347-020-00190-3] [PMID: 33501372]

[10]　Mosnaim GS, Stempel H, Van Sickle D, Stempel DA. The adoption and implementation of digital health care in the post COVID–19 era. J Allergy Clin Immunol Pract 2020; 8(8): 2484-6.
[http://dx.doi.org/10.1016/j.jaip.2020.06.006] [PMID: 32585407]

[11]　Yang T, Duncan TV. Challenges and potential solutions for nanosensors intended for use with foods. Nat Nanotechnol 2021; 16(3): 251-65.
[http://dx.doi.org/10.1038/s41565-021-00867-7] [PMID: 33712739]

[12]　Kirilov N. Capture of real-time data from electronic health records: scenarios and solutions. mHealth 2024; 10: 14.
[http://dx.doi.org/10.21037/mhealth-24-2] [PMID: 38689616]

[13]　Huang C, Koppel R, McGreevey JD III, Craven CK, Schreiber R. Transitions from one electronic health record to another: challenges, pitfalls, and recommendations. Appl Clin Inform 2020; 11(5): 742-54.
[http://dx.doi.org/10.1055/s-0040-1718535] [PMID: 33176389]

[14]　Haleem A, Javaid M, Pratap Singh R, Suman R. Medical 4.0 technologies for healthcare: Features, capabilities, and applications. Inter Things Cyber-Phys Sys 2022; 2: 12-30.
[http://dx.doi.org/10.1016/j.iotcps.2022.04.001]

[15]　Khatiwada P, Yang B, Lin JC, Blobel B. Patient-Generated Health Data (PGHD): Understanding, Requirements, Challenges, and Existing Techniques for Data Security and Privacy. J Pers Med 2024; 14(3): 282.
[http://dx.doi.org/10.3390/jpm14030282] [PMID: 38541024]

[16]　Krzyszczyk P, Acevedo A, Davidoff EJ, *et al.*, The growing role of precision and personalised medicine for cancer treatment. Technology. 2018 Sep 11;6(03n04):79-100.

[17]　Jain AK, Jain S. Understanding organisational culture and leadership-enhance efficiency and productivity. Pranjana. Pranjana J Manag Aware 2013; 16(2): 43-53.

[18]　Kumar P. Managing service flexibility in healthcare for improved customer experience: a data-driven approach. J Strateg Mark 2024; 32(7): 891-912.
[http://dx.doi.org/10.1080/0965254X.2022.2096671]

[19]　Zeb S, Fnu N, Abbasi N, Fahad M. AI in healthcare: revolutionising diagnosis and therapy. Intl J Multidis Sci Arts 2024; 3(3): 118-28.
[http://dx.doi.org/10.47709/ijmdsa.v3i3.4546]

[20]　Naithani K, Tiwari S, Chauhan AS, Wadawadagi RS. Smart health revolution: unleashing the power of AI, electronic health records and the IoT for sustainable systems. In: Kumar A, Sharma R, Dey N, Eds. Big data analytics and intelligent applications for smart and secure healthcare services. 1st ed. Boca Raton (FL): CRC Press 2025; p. 28.

[21]　Alrahbi D, Khan M, Hussain M. Exploring the motivators of technology adoption in healthcare. Int J Healthc Manag 2021; 14(1): 50-63.
[http://dx.doi.org/10.1080/20479700.2019.1607451]

[22]　Nusem E, Straker K, Wrigley C. Design innovation for health and medicine. Singapore: Palgrave Macmillan; 2020 Jan 1.
[http://dx.doi.org/10.1007/978-981-15-4362-3]

[23]　Warner JJ, Benjamin IJ, Churchwell K, *et al.* Advancing healthcare reform: the American Heart Association's 2020 statement of principles for adequate, accessible, and affordable health care: a presidential advisory from the American Heart Association. Circulation 2020; 141(10): e601-14.
[http://dx.doi.org/10.1161/CIR.0000000000000759] [PMID: 32008369]

[24]　Almeida J, Farias J, Carvalho H. Drivers of the technology adoption in healthcare. BBR. Brazilian Business Review 2017; 14(3): 336-51.
[http://dx.doi.org/10.15728/bbr.2017.14.3.5]

[25] Oyeniyi J. The role of AI and mobile apps in patient-centric healthcare delivery. World J Adv Res Rev 2024; 22(1): 1897-907.
[http://dx.doi.org/10.30574/wjarr.2024.22.1.1331]

[26] Alotaibi YK, Federico F. The impact of health information technology on patient safety. Saudi Med J 2017; 38(12): 1173-80.
[http://dx.doi.org/10.15537/smj.2017.12.20631] [PMID: 29209664]

[27] Booth RG, Strudwick G, McBride S, O'Connor S, López AL. How the nursing profession should adapt for a digital future. BMJ 2021; 373: n1190.

[28] Alhomiany AM, Alsharif MZ, ALsolumany FJ, et al. Transforming healthcare through effective health administration practices: a systematic review. J Ecohuman 2024; 3(7): 2708-16.

[29] Rindfleisch TC. Privacy, information technology, and health care. Commun ACM 1997; 40(8): 92-100.
[http://dx.doi.org/10.1145/257874.257896]

[30] Hussain S, Mubeen I, Ullah N, *et al.* Modern diagnostic imaging technique applications and risk factors in the medical field: a review. BioMed Res Intl 2022; 2022(1): 5164970.
[http://dx.doi.org/10.1155/2022/5164970]

[31] Poudel A, Nissen L. Telepharmacy: a pharmacist's perspective on the clinical benefits and challenges. Integr Pharm Res Pract 2016; 5: 75-82.
[http://dx.doi.org/10.2147/IPRP.S101685] [PMID: 29354542]

[32] Tokuç B, Varol G. Medical education in the era of advancing technology. Balkan Med J 2023; 40(6): 395-9.
[http://dx.doi.org/10.4274/balkanmedj.galenos.2023.2023-7-79] [PMID: 37706676]

[33] Øvretveit J, Scott T, Rundall TG, Shortell SM, Brommels M. Improving quality through effective healthcare information technology implementation. Int J Qual Health Care 2007; 19(5): 259-66.
[http://dx.doi.org/10.1093/intqhc/mzm031] [PMID: 17717038]

[34] Winman T, Rystedt H. Electronic patient records in action. Health Informatics J 2011; 17(1): 51-62.
[http://dx.doi.org/10.1177/1460458210396330] [PMID: 25133770]

[35] Monteiro AC, França RP, Estrela VV, Iano Y, Khelassi A, Razmjooy N. Health 4.0: applications, management, technologies and review. Med Tech J 2018; 2(4): 262-76.

[36] Adeghe EP, Okolo CA, Ojeyinka OT. A review of emerging trends in telemedicine: Healthcare delivery transformations. Int J Life Sci Res Arch 2024; 6(1): 137-47.
[http://dx.doi.org/10.53771/ijlsra.2024.6.1.0040]

[37] Malasinghe LP, Ramzan N, Dahal K. Remote patient monitoring: a comprehensive study. J Ambient Intell Humaniz Comput 2019; 10(1): 57-76.
[http://dx.doi.org/10.1007/s12652-017-0598-x]

[38] Krishnan G, Singh S, Pathania M, *et al.* Artificial intelligence in clinical medicine: catalyzing a sustainable global healthcare paradigm. Front Artif Intel 2023; 6: 1227091.
[http://dx.doi.org/10.3389/frai.2023.1227091] [PMID: 37705603]

[39] Ahmed Z, Mohamed K, Zeeshan S, Dong X. Artificial intelligence with multi-functional machine learning platform development for better healthcare and precision medicine. Database (Oxford) 2020; 2020: baaa010.
[http://dx.doi.org/10.1093/database/baaa010] [PMID: 32185396]

[40] Ibrahim T, Ali H. The impact of wearable IoT devices on early disease detection and prevention. Int J App Heal Care Ana 2023; 8(8): 1-5.

[41] Del-Valle-Soto C, López-Pimentel JC, Vázquez-Castillo J, *et al.* A comprehensive review of behavior change techniques in wearables and IoT: implications for health and well-being. Sensors (Basel) 2024; 24(8): 2429.

[http://dx.doi.org/10.3390/s24082429] [PMID: 38676044]

[42] Khatri S, Alzahrani FA, Ansari MTJ, Agrawal A, Kumar R, Khan RA. A systematic analysis on blockchain integration with healthcare domain: scope and challenges. IEEE Access 2021; 9: 84666-87. [http://dx.doi.org/10.1109/ACCESS.2021.3087608]

[43] Sharma DS, Chaturvedi R. Blockchain technology in healthcare billing: enhancing transparency and Security. Int J Res Public Sem 2017; 10(2): 106-117.

[44] Ibeh CV, Elufioye OA, Olorunsogo T, Asuzu OF, Nduubuisi NL, Daraojimba AI. Data analytics in healthcare: a review of patient-centric approaches and healthcare delivery. World J Adv Res Rev 2024; 21(2): 1750–1760. [http://dx.doi.org/10.30574/wjarr.2024.21.2.0246]

[45] Choudhary V, Mehta A, Patel K, Niaz M, Panwala M, Nwagwu U. Integrating data analytics and decision support systems in public health management. South East Euro J Pub Heal 2024; 1: pp. 158-72.

[46] Zakerabasali S, Ayyoubzadeh SM, Baniasadi T, Yazdani A, Abhari S. Mobile health technology and healthcare providers: systemic barriers to adoption. Healthc Inform Res 2021; 27(4): 267-78. [http://dx.doi.org/10.4258/hir.2021.27.4.267] [PMID: 34788907]

[47] Machireddy JR. Revolutionizing Claims Processing in the Healthcare Industry: The Expanding Role of Automation and AI. Hong Kong J AI Med 2022; 2(1): 10-36.

[48] Petersson L, Larsson I, Nygren JM, *et al.* Challenges to implementing artificial intelligence in healthcare: a qualitative interview study with healthcare leaders in Sweden. BMC Health Serv Res 2022; 22(1): 850. [http://dx.doi.org/10.1186/s12913-022-08215-8] [PMID: 35778736]

[49] Zatini G, Della Porta A, Za S. Deciphering barriers and strategies in environmental management accounting (EMA) adoption: a comprehensive two-decade analysis. Corp Soc Respon Envir Manag 2025 May; 32(3): 3355-70. [http://dx.doi.org/10.1002/csr.3130]

[50] Suryanti R, Mardiharini M, Kisworo AN, Untari FD. Improving the sustainability of silage adoption in dairy cattle farming: analysis of determining factors and strategies for increasing farm capacity. J Penyuluhan Pertanian 2025 May 29; 20(1): 14-28. [http://dx.doi.org/10.51852/7eayjd09]

[51] Markaki A, Malhotra S, Billings R, Theus L. Training needs assessment: tool utilization and global impact. BMC Med Educ 2021; 21(1): 310. [http://dx.doi.org/10.1186/s12909-021-02748-y] [PMID: 34059018]

[52] Sanghi S. The handbook of competency mapping: understanding, designing and implementing competency models in organisations. New Delhi: SAGE Publications 2003; p. 142.

[53] Gaspard J, Yang CM. Training needs assessment of health care professionals in a developing country: the example of Saint Lucia. BMC Med Educ 2016; 16(1): 112. [http://dx.doi.org/10.1186/s12909-016-0638-9] [PMID: 27116929]

[54] Mormina M, Pinder S. A conceptual framework for the training of trainers (ToT) interventions in global health. Global Health. 2018 Oct 22; 14(1): 100.

[55] Kapoor C, Solomon N. Understanding and managing generational differences in the workplace. Worldw Hosp Tour Themes 2011; 3(4): 308-18. [http://dx.doi.org/10.1108/17554211111162435]

[56] Sharma S, Rawal R, Shah D. Addressing the challenges of AI-based telemedicine: Best practices and lessons learned. J Educ Health Promot 2023; 12(1): 338. [http://dx.doi.org/10.4103/jehp.jehp_402_23] [PMID: 38023098]

[57] Noe RA, Tews MJ. Strategic training and development. In: Boxall P, Purcell J, Wright PM, Eds. The

Routledge companion to strategic human resource management. 1st ed. London: Routledge 2008; p. 23.
[http://dx.doi.org/10.4324/9780203889015.ch16]

[58] Islam Z, Pollock K, Patterson A, *et al.* Thinking ahead about medical treatments in advanced illness: a qualitative study of barriers and enablers in end-of-life care planning with patients and families from ethnically diverse backgrounds. Heal Soc Care Del Res 2023; 11(7): 1-135.
[http://dx.doi.org/10.3310/JVFW4781] [PMID: 37464868]

[59] Kalyani LK. The role of technology in education: Enhancing learning outcomes and 21st century skills. Int J Sci Res Mod Sci Tech 2024 Apr 11; 3(4): 5-10.

[60] Marougkas A, Troussas C, Krouska A, Sgouropoulou C. Virtual reality in education: a review of learning theories, approaches and methodologies for the last decade. Electronics (Basel) 2023; 12(13): 2832.
[http://dx.doi.org/10.3390/electronics12132832]

[61] Chen Z, Liang N, Zhang H, *et al.* Harnessing the power of clinical decision support systems: challenges and opportunities. Open Heart 2023; 10(2): e002432.
[http://dx.doi.org/10.1136/openhrt-2023-002432] [PMID: 38016787]

[62] Regan EA, Agha AM, Brookshire RG. Digital learning in healthcare: where we are and where we are going. In: Mulder RH, Beausaert S, Schaffar B, Eds. The SAGE handbook of learning and work. London: SAGE 2022; pp. 311-328.

[63] Badea DO, Darabont DC, Chis TV, Trifu A. The transformative impact of E-learning on workplace safety and health training in the industry: A comprehensive analysis of effectiveness, implementation, and future opportunities. Int J Educ Inf Technol 2024; 18: 105-18.
[http://dx.doi.org/10.46300/9109.2024.18.11]

[64] Tang YM, Chau KY, Kwok APK, Zhu T, Ma X. A systematic review of immersive technology applications for medical practice and education - Trends, application areas, recipients, teaching contents, evaluation methods, and performance. Educ Res Rev 2022; 35: 100429.
[http://dx.doi.org/10.1016/j.edurev.2021.100429]

[65] Ahmad A, Desouza KC, Maynard SB, Naseer H, Baskerville RL. How integration of cyber security management and incident response enables organizational learning. J Assoc Inf Sci Technol 2020; 71(8): 939-53.
[http://dx.doi.org/10.1002/asi.24311]

[66] Brown S, Gommers J, Serrano O. From cyber security information sharing to threat management. Proceedings of the 2nd ACM workshop on information sharing and collaborative security 2015; 43-9.
[http://dx.doi.org/10.1145/2808128.2808133]

[67] Tene T, Vique López DF, Valverde Aguirre PE, Orna Puente LM, Vacacela Gomez C. Virtual reality and augmented reality in medical education: an umbrella review. Frontiers in Digital Health 2024; 6: 1365345.
[http://dx.doi.org/10.3389/fdgth.2024.1365345] [PMID: 38550715]

[68] Bhati D, Deogade MS, Kanyal D. Improving patient outcomes through effective hospital administration: a comprehensive review. Cureus 2023; 15(10): e47731.
[http://dx.doi.org/10.7759/cureus.47731] [PMID: 38021686]

[69] Strielkowski W, Grebennikova V, Lisovskiy A, Rakhimova G, Vasileva T. AI-driven adaptive learning for sustainable educational transformation. Sustainable Development. 2025 Apr; 33(2): 1921-47.
[http://dx.doi.org/10.1002/sd.3221]

[70] Pizzuti C, Palmieri C, Shaw T. The role of medical regulations and medical regulators in fostering the use of eHealth data for strengthened continuing professional development (CPD): a document analysis with key informants' interviews. BMC Medical Education. 2025 Jul 1; 25(1): 871.
[http://dx.doi.org/10.1186/s12909-025-07443-w]

[71] Dubois CA, Singh D. From staff-mix to skill-mix and beyond: towards a systemic approach to health workforce management. Hum Resour Health 2009; 7(1): 87.
[http://dx.doi.org/10.1186/1478-4491-7-87] [PMID: 20021682]

[72] Needleman J, Hassmiller S. The role of nurses in improving hospital quality and efficiency: real-world results. Health Aff (Millwood) 2009; 28 (Suppl. 3): w625-33.
[http://dx.doi.org/10.1377/hlthaff.28.4.w625]

[73] McCuaig L, Hay P. Overcoming barriers and problem solving. In: Brown T, Macdonald D, Wright J, Eds. The future of health, wellbeing and physical education. Cham: Palgrave Macmillan 2016; pp. 135-148.
[http://dx.doi.org/10.1007/978-3-319-31667-3_10]

[74] McPake B, Witter S, Ensor T, *et al.* Removing financial barriers to access reproductive, maternal and newborn health services: the challenges and policy implications for human resources for health. Hum Resour Health 2013; 11(1): 46.
[http://dx.doi.org/10.1186/1478-4491-11-46] [PMID: 24053731]

[75] Buchanan DA, Denyer D, Jaina J, *et al.* How do they manage? A qualitative study of the realities of middle and front-line management work in health care. Health Serv Deliv Res 2013; 1(4): 1-248.
[http://dx.doi.org/10.3310/hsdr01040] [PMID: 25642544]

[76] Lilly CL, Bryant LL, Leary JM, *et al.* Evaluation of the effectiveness of a problem-solving intervention addressing barriers to cardiovascular disease prevention behaviors in 3 underserved populations: Colorado, North Carolina, West Virginia, 2009. Prev Chronic Dis 2014; 11: 130249.
[http://dx.doi.org/10.5888/pcd11.130249] [PMID: 24602586]

[77] Cresswell KM, Bates DW, Sheikh A. Ten key considerations for the successful implementation and adoption of large-scale health information technology. J Am Med Inform Assoc 2013; 20(e1): e9-e13.
[http://dx.doi.org/10.1136/amiajnl-2013-001684] [PMID: 23599226]

[78] Huang E, Chang CC. Case studies of implementation of interactive e-health tools on hospital websites. E-Service Journal. 2014 Jan 1;9(2):46-61.

[79] Abdul S, Adeghe EP, Adegoke BO, Adegoke AA, Udedeh EH. Public-private partnerships in health sector innovation: Lessons from around the world. Magn Sci Adv Biol Pharm 2024; 12(1): 45-59.

[80] Kala ESM. Challenges of technology in African countries: a case sudy of Zambia. Open J Saf Sci Tech 2023; 13(4): 202-30.
[http://dx.doi.org/10.4236/ojsst.2023.134011]

[81] Akingbola A, Adegbesan A, Ojo O, Otumara JU, Alao UH. Artificial intelligence and cancer care in Africa. Journal of Medicine, Surgery, and Public Health 2024; 3: 100132.
[http://dx.doi.org/10.1016/j.glmedi.2024.100132]

[82] Hennessy S, D'Angelo S, McIntyre N, *et al.* Technology used for teacher professional development in low and middle-income countries: A systematic review. Computers and Education Open 2022; 3: 100080.
[http://dx.doi.org/10.1016/j.caeo.2022.100080]

[83] Foo CD, Shrestha P, Wang L, *et al.* Integrating tuberculosis and noncommunicable diseases care in low- and middle-income countries (LMICs): A systematic review. PLoS Med 2022; 19(1): e1003899.
[http://dx.doi.org/10.1371/journal.pmed.1003899] [PMID: 35041654]

[84] Subbaraman R, de Mondesert L, Musiimenta A, *et al.* Digital adherence technologies for the management of tuberculosis therapy: mapping the landscape and research priorities. BMJ Glob Health 2018; 3(5): e001018.
[http://dx.doi.org/10.1136/bmjgh-2018-001018] [PMID: 30364330]

[85] Berkhout F, Hertin J. De-materialising and re-materialising: digital technologies and the environment. Futures 2004; 36(8): 903-20.
[http://dx.doi.org/10.1016/j.futures.2004.01.003]

[86]   Deen J, Mengel MA, Clemens JD. Epidemiology of cholera. Vaccine 2020; 38 (Suppl. 1): A31-40.
[http://dx.doi.org/10.1016/j.vaccine.2019.07.078] [PMID: 31395455]

[87]   Phan JM, Kim S, Linh ĐTT, Cosimi LA, Pollack TM. Telehealth interventions for HIV in low-and
middle-income countries. Curr HIV/AIDS Rep 2022; 19(6): 600-9.
[http://dx.doi.org/10.1007/s11904-022-00630-0] [PMID: 36156183]

[88]   ElKefi S, Asan O. How technology impacts communication between cancer patients and their health
care providers: A systematic literature review. Int J Med Inform 2021; 149: 104430.
[http://dx.doi.org/10.1016/j.ijmedinf.2021.104430] [PMID: 33684711]

[89]   Mattison G, Canfell O, Forrester D, *et al.* The influence of wearables on health care outcomes in
chronic disease: systematic review. J Med Internet Res 2022; 24(7): e36690.
[http://dx.doi.org/10.2196/36690] [PMID: 35776492]

[90]   Sommer AC, Blumenthal EZ. Telemedicine in ophthalmology in view of the emerging COVID-19
outbreak. Graefes Arch Clin Exp Ophthalmol 2020; 258(11): 2341-52.
[http://dx.doi.org/10.1007/s00417-020-04879-2] [PMID: 32813110]

[91]   Nygård HT, Nguyen L, Berg RC. Effect of remote patient monitoring for patients with chronic kidney
disease who perform dialysis at home: a systematic review. BMJ Open 2022; 12(12): e061772.
[http://dx.doi.org/10.1136/bmjopen-2022-061772] [PMID: 36600376]

[92]   Ronco C, Crepaldi C, Rosner MH, Eds. Remote patient management in peritoneal dialysis. Basel:
Karger; 2019. [http://dx.doi.org/10.1159/000496317]

[93]   Talbot B, Farnbach S, Tong A, *et al.* Patient and clinician perspectives on remote patient monitoring in
peritoneal dialysis. Can J Kidney Health Dis 2022; 9: 20543581221084499.
[http://dx.doi.org/10.1177/20543581221084499] [PMID: 35340772]

[94]   Bajwa M. Emerging 21st century medical technologies. Pak J Med Sci 2014; 30(3): 649-55.
[PMID: 24948997]

[95]   Wang Q, Su M, Zhang M, Li R. Integrating digital technologies and public health to fight Covid-19
pandemic: key technologies, applications, challenges and outlook of digital healthcare. Int J Environ
Res Public Health 2021; 18(11): 6053.
[http://dx.doi.org/10.3390/ijerph18116053] [PMID: 34199831]

[96]   Basulo-Ribeiro J, Teixeira L. The future of healthcare with industry 5.0: Preliminary interview-based
qualitative analysis. Future Internet 2024; 16(3): 68.
[http://dx.doi.org/10.3390/fi16030068]

[97]   Iqbal M. AI in education: Personalized learning and adaptive assessment. Cosm Bull Bus Manag 2023;
2(1): 280-97.

[98]   Shanthi D, Ashok G, Biswal C, Udharika S, Varshini S, Sindhu G. Ai-driven adaptive it training: A
personalized learning framework for enhanced knowledge retention and engagement. Met Mater Eng
2025 May 7; 31(5): 136-45. [https://doi.org/10.63278/mme.vi.1567]

[99]   Junaid SB, Imam AA, Balogun AO, et al. Recent advancements in emerging technologies for
healthcare management systems: a survey. Healthcare (Basel). 2022 Oct 3; 10(10): 1940. [doi:
10.3390/healthcare10101940]

[100] Frehywot S, Vovides Y, Talib Z, *et al.* E-learning in medical education in resource constrained low-
and middle-income countries. Hum Resour Health 2013; 11(1): 4.
[http://dx.doi.org/10.1186/1478-4491-11-4] [PMID: 23379467]

[101] Shahriar SHB, Arafat S, Islam I, *et al.* The emergence of e-learning and online-based training during
the COVID-19 crisis: an exploratory investigation from Bangladesh. Management Matters 2023;
20(1): 1-15.
[http://dx.doi.org/10.1108/MANM-01-2022-0007]

[102] Singh J, Steele K, Singh L. Combining the best of online and face-to-face learning: Hybrid and

blended learning approach for COVID-19, post-vaccine, & post-pandemic world. J Educ Technol Syst 2021; 50(2): 140-71.
[http://dx.doi.org/10.1177/00472395211047865]

[103] Elendu C, Amaechi DC, Okatta AU, *et al.* The impact of simulation-based training in medical education: A review. Medicine (Baltimore) 2024; 103(27): e38813.
[http://dx.doi.org/10.1097/MD.0000000000038813] [PMID: 38968472]

SUBJECT INDEX

A

Accessibility 1, 2, 3, 11, 13, 17, 19, 20, 22, 24, 64, 65, 71, 80, 88, 90, 91, 99, 113, 117, 120, 130, 138, 140, 145, 147, 162, 164, 165, 168, 174
Accountable care organizations 143, 151
Advancements in mobile devices 1
Affordability 2, 24, 117, 138, 139, 140, 145, 153
AI assistants 1
AI-driven scheduling 42
AIDS 174, 175
Arthritis 175
Artificial intelligence 2, 8, 10, 12, 34, 64, 78, 88, 89, 145, 161, 162
Asthma 14, 16
Augmented reality 96
Automation and workflow optimisation 47

B

Big data 6
Billing and invoicing 40
Biometric scanners 38
Biosensors 9, 163
Blindness 175
Blockchain 32, 41, 43, 44, 55, 56, 64, 131, 152, 168
Blood pressure 2, 6, 10, 45, 104, 118, 123, 167
Bluetooth 9
Budget monitoring 151
Bundled payments 138, 143, 153

C

Cancer management 14, 15
Capitation and global budgets 144
Caregiving robots 93
Cholera 175

Chronic

Chronic 1, 2, 10, 13, 20, 21, 24, 75, 79, 104, 114, 115, 116, 118, 120, 122, 123, 128, 129, 131, 145, 167, 175
conditions 2, 10, 20, 75, 79, 104, 118, 120, 128, 145, 167
diseases 1, 10, 13, 21, 24, 75, 79, 114, 115, 116, 122, 123, 129, 131, 167, 175
Clinical decision support systems 72
Clinical document architecture 52
Cloud computing 2, 32, 46, 47, 64, 95, 100
Cloud infrastructure 11
Cloud-based software 46
Cognitive behavioural therapy 8, 17
Community health workers 174
Continuity of care document 71
Cost-effective platform 1
COVID-19 pandemic 8, 69, 122, 175
Cross-department collaboration 50
Cultural stigmas 4
Cybersecurity 33, 53

D

Da vinci surgical system 101
Data 52, 53, 73, 74, 77, 88
exchange services 73
exchange standards 52
privacy and security 77
repositories 73
security 53, 64, 88
Decision-making 2, 6, 8, 21, 33, 36, 39, 42, 47, 49, 50, 78, 91, 96, 100, 123, 148, 150, 153, 161, 166, 168, 171, 172
Decision-support apps 8
Deep learning algorithms 9
Diagnostic precision 2
Digital 1, 2, 4, 23, 124, 126, 131, 139, 145, 164, 178
health records 1
literacy 4, 23, 124, 126, 131, 164, 178
payment solutions 139, 145
transformation 2

www.ingramcontent.com/pod-product-compliance
Lightning Source LLC
Chambersburg PA
CBHW080020240326
41598CB00075B/477